Contents

About the author

Marina Lewycka is a lecturer and freelance writer. She contributed to the BBC handbook *Who Cares Now?* and her training resource pack *Survival Skills for Carers* is published by the National Extension College with support from the Department of Health. She has been involved in the organisation of weekend courses for carers. Marina is also the author of four other books in the 'Carers Handbook' series.

Acknowledgements

I would like to thank all the people who have contributed their knowledge and experience to help make this book. I would especially like to thank the members of the Sheffield Hard of Hearing Club and the Chesterfield Lipreading Group who provided many of the personal accounts which bring the book to life, also Judith Sutton, Margaret Miller and Pat Crabtree. Many thanks to the Sheffield Deaf Club for permission to quote from their book *Read My Lips, Hear My Hands*. I would also like to thank Maureen Bagley, Martha Moyses and Steve Creswell of Sheffield Social Services, Jackie Gill of the Royal Hallamshire Hospital Audiology Clinic and Val Rose of the British Tinnitus Association for their help and encouragement.

I would particularly like to acknowledge the contribution of Christine Wright, lipreading teacher and chair of the Sheffield Hard of Hearing Club, for her unstintingly generous support and patience, without which this book would have been much poorer.

Finally, thanks are due to Anne Hodgson, Philippa Smart and their colleagues at The Royal National Institute for Deaf People (RNID); Richard Holloway of Age Concern England who helped initiate this book, and Vinnette Marshall and Marion Peat for their help in production of the text.

Introduction

When I told friends that I was writing a book about hearing loss, quite a few of them responded by cupping a hand behind their ear and asking, 'You what?' In our society, hearing loss is still widely regarded as something we can joke about.

For the one in seven people in Britain who have a hearing loss, their disability is no joke. Talking and listening to people is still the main way we communicate. Losing that ability can mean slipping into a world of isolation and loneliness. People with hearing loss have to deal both with their disability and with society's attitude towards them.

But it doesn't have to be like this. There are many ways in which people can be helped to communicate, however severe their hearing loss. From hearing aids to hearing dogs, from lipreading to induction loops, this book explores the technology, the communication techniques and the social support available to someone with hearing loss. It is full of practical advice and information about how you can help someone to make the most of the hearing that they have.

If you are a carer living with or supporting someone with a hearing loss, there are aids and devices you can get, techniques you can learn, people you can call on, to help open up the whole world of communication to them.

Throughout the book, deaf and hard of hearing people, people with related conditions such as tinnitus, and carers, speak out about their experiences and frustrations. They share the skills and insights they have learned about managing in a hearing world.

1 Coming to terms with hearing loss

It is hard for someone who has not lost their hearing to imagine the feelings of isolation and despair that can engulf someone who realises they are going deaf. We can all feel sympathy for a blind person whose impairment cuts them off from the beauty of the natural world, but hearing loss, which cuts someone off from human society, is still treated as something of a joke. The elderly aunt with the ear trumpet, the granddad who is 'selectively deaf' and 'only hears when he wants to', these are stereotypes which can still raise a smile, even in our so-called enlightened times.

People who are born deaf, or lose their hearing while they are young, may well have built their own society in the Deaf Community based on communication through sign language. But someone who has lived in the hearing community for most of their life, then loses their hearing in later life, may feel they have no place where they fit in.

If the person you care for has lost or is losing their hearing, it is important that you understand how they may be feeling, so that you can work with them to find solutions.

Joan

'When I first met Harry nearly 20 years ago I had no experience of deafness or deaf people. I didn't realise he was deaf at first – he's very clever at covering it up – and by the time I realised, it didn't make any difference. The language of love doesn't need any words – we managed!

'Then I realised that if we were going to be together, we would have to learn how to communicate. We joined the Hard of Hearing Club, and went to lipreading classes together. I learnt fingerspelling and lipspeaking, too. That was wonderful, because we met many other people in the same position.

'I'm a singer, and I really appreciate it that he always comes with me, and works the PA system, even though he doesn't enjoy music much. We have a lot of fun together. We've been very lucky.'

Harry

'I had a perforated eardrum through scarlet fever and I shouldn't really have been in the RAF at all, but I didn't tell them. In the RAF I was subjected to a lot of noise, and now I only have 25 per cent hearing in my good ear, and they tell me the eardrum is very thin and could go at any time.

'When I first went deaf I felt very isolated. I lost all my confidence. I found myself opting out of things. Going to lipreading classes with Joan has given me back my confidence. Now we're learning sign language, in case my hearing goes altogether.'

Feelings about hearing loss

Our society is based on communication. Someone who suddenly or gradually loses their ability to communicate may feel upset, angry, stupid, embarrassed, isolated, depressed, frustrated, or a mixture of all these. Some people with hearing loss explain it below in their own words.

Chris

'As a child I always had appallingly smelly ears. I remember being very embarrassed about it. I vividly remember going to the school clinic three times a week for ear drops and having very frequent ear syringes. When I was 17 I had further treatment, and again at 22. I was then working in an all-male environment, training to be a chartered accountant. I went for my hospital appointment and was told I would probably need a hearing aid in the future. I was devastated. I walked around town sobbing for nearly an hour before I was composed enough to go back to work.

'For years I was very embarrassed about my hearing problem and tried to hide it. I gave up Sunday School teaching and some of my Boys' Brigade work because I couldn't follow what the children were saying and hear all their quips.

'There's a lot of situations in which I feel stupid, or I feel I have to apologise because I haven't understood someone. The thing that hurts most is when people pretend it's a joke, cupping their hand behind their ear and saying "Pardon?" Or if you ask someone to repeat something because you didn't hear, and they say, "Oh, it doesn't matter."'

Freda

'Most of the time people are not aware, unless you are "visibly deaf". Even people who know we are deaf just forget most of the time. We have to keep on reminding them. I wish people could be more patient – accept what has happened and be supportive. I suppose it's something we have to live with.'

Albert

'If you're finding it frustrating trying to talk to someone with hearing loss, try to remember it's just as bad for them!'

Learning to accept hearing loss

Whether it happens suddenly or over a period of time, losing one's hearing can come as a terrible blow. Do not expect the person you care for to accept their new situation and adapt overnight, or even over months. Many people go through a period of mourning while they come to terms with their loss.

The charity Hearing Concern has a network of trained advisers, who are usually people with a hearing loss themselves, who understand the feelings of someone who has lost or is losing their hearing. They can visit someone at home, and give them personal, friendly and sympathetic support, to help them come to terms with their loss. They can advise about practical aspects of communication, but more importantly they can help someone who has just lost their hearing to feel better and more optimistic about their future as a person with a hearing loss. See page 140 for Hearing Concern contact details.

Chris

'What changed my life was when I gave up accountancy and retrained as a lipreading teacher. Then I went on to become a Hearing Concern volunteer adviser. That was directly as a result of my own hearing loss. My whole life changed. Now I've become much more confident and outgoing about hearing loss, because I am speaking up for all hard of hearing people, not just for myself.'

However, some people are reluctant to discuss their feelings and anxieties with a stranger. If the person you care for does not want to ask for help, do not press them, but you yourself might find it helpful to discuss ways of adjusting to hearing loss, so you can give them better support.

How the carer can help

You can help the person you care for to come to terms with their hearing loss by learning about deafness and hearing loss, and finding out information that will be useful to them:

- Learn about hearing loss, especially the type of hearing loss experienced by the person you care for, and find out what aids and treatments may be available.
- Find out how the person you care for prefers to communicate, and try to learn new communication techniques, such as lip-speaking or sign language. Encourage them by going along to lipreading or sign language classes with them (see pages 28–30).
- Encourage the person you care for to have a hearing test, and find out about different types of hearing aids.
- Talk to the person you care for about their changing needs, and discuss ways in which they will be able to manage every-day situations at home. Send off for the free RNID Sound Advantage *Solutions* catalogue (details on page 67), and discuss aids and equipment which they would find helpful. (See Chapters 5 and 6 for more about managing at home.)
- Become more 'deaf aware' yourself so you can help and speak up for the person you care for when you go out together.

Note **Remember, the person you care for may not be feeling very motivated at this point, so you can help by doing some of the legwork or some of the telephoning around, and you can help them feel less isolated by showing interest and being positive about the future.**

Pauline

'Mum went deaf as we were growing up, so Dad looked after us a lot. She couldn't hear us, so she never got up with us in the night. Poor old Dad, he often looked like a zombie in the mornings. But he was always very supportive. He would write things down for Mum. Now my sister and I take notes for her.

'I would say Mum's deafness has brought us closer as a family, and has opened up new doors for us. I'm now at College doing the first year of a degree. I've also been running some training in deaf awareness, and I would like to train as a sign language interpreter.'

Hearing loss and relationships

Hearing loss can have a profound effect on personal relationships. Breakdown of communication can lead to friction, whether it is in the big world of politics or in the close world of families. This is something people with hearing loss know only too well.

Chris

'Arguments occur because of misunderstandings. Friction occurs when people forget, and speak from another room, or with their back turned. I know I cause annoyance when I'm watching TV with the loop on, because my family speak to me, and I don't reply. I've known divorces occur directly because of deafness.'

Joan

'We've been together nearly 20 years, but sometimes I still forget and start talking as if he was a hearing person, and tempers flare.'

Albert

'Hearing loss causes a lot of problems in families – people just get irritated with each other. Someone talks to you, and you don't reply, and they think, "Oh, he's just being bloody-minded."

'The need to constantly ask people to repeat a conversation can lead to frustration and isolation. Do you create a situation where you're being difficult, or do you just opt out? Sometimes, it seems as though it's just too much bother to try to communicate. In my case, I think it led to the breakdown of my marriage.'

A partner or relative of someone with hearing loss may need to be particularly understanding and easy-going to always give support, and never allow bad feeling or irritation to develop. Of course you would have to be superhuman to achieve this all the time, but it is worth making the effort. The more supportive you can be, the more the person you care for will regain their self-confidence and independence.

Rene

'My mother died when I was 19, and later, I realised I couldn't hear so well. People said, "It's the shock, and being so upset. It will get better soon." But it didn't. Our family GP sent me to the hospital, where they did their best, but it wasn't much help to me. At this time, I was very low in spirit.

'I was 21 when I met the young good-looking lad that I married in 1949. This year we celebrated our Golden Wedding. I had two sons, learned to drive a car, learned dressmaking, took classes in pottery and flower arranging, worked at the checkout in a supermarket, and later in our own grocery business.

'It is him that gave me the support, encouragement and confidence all through my life.'

Signs of deafness

The classic sign of deafness is when someone has the television turned up so loud it is annoying to other people. Or they may think everyone else is mumbling, because they have lost their hearing at the higher frequencies, so consonant sounds are not clear.

Albert

'I first realised I was going deaf when people in the office told me I was shouting down the phone.'

Gillian

'I didn't want to believe I was going deaf. I blamed people in my family for mumbling, or whispering.'

If the person you care for has one or more of these signs, you should try to persuade them to have their hearing assessed:

- has the television turned up very loud;
- often asks people to repeat what they said;
- shouts when on the telephone;
- doesn't answer the telephone or the doorbell;
- complains that other people mumble;
- doesn't join in conversation when in a group of people;
- can't tell which direction a sound is coming from;
- seems to give inappropriate responses in conversation;
- can't follow conversation in noisy places such as pubs or restaurants.

Having your hearing tested

Don't be surprised if the person you care for seems to be reluctant to go for a hearing test. If they are still managing to cope with their increasing hearing problem, they may not be ready to admit that it has got to the stage where they need to do something about it.

Arnold

'Eventually I plucked up the courage to get my hearing assessed. I was embarrassed about getting a hearing aid, because I thought it was a stigma to have a hearing loss.

'When I first got my hearing aid, I would not wear it outside because I didn't want people to know.'

Don't put it off!

There are good reasons for someone having their hearing tested sooner rather than later. There is plenty of evidence that the older a person is, the harder they find it to get used to using a hearing aid. On the positive side, the sooner they get used to their hearing aid, the sooner they will find themselves able to join in and enjoy conversation again.

Another reason for not putting it off is that there could be a waiting list of several months for the first hospital appointment.

The first step in hearing assessment is to see the doctor, who will check the ears, and decide whether the person needs to see a specialist (there is more about this on page 10). When they have crossed this hurdle, they may still have a long wait for their first hearing test.

Be persistent

You may need to use all your powers of persuasion at this stage, as, sadly, some GPs still regard hearing loss as a natural part of ageing, and therefore not something that should be treated.

In fact there is much that can be done to lessen the effects of hearing loss. Having a hearing aid fitted can have quite a dramatic effect on someone's life (see Chapter 4). In addition, the GP may also refer your relative for hearing therapy. Some of the equipment described in Chapter 5 may also be available from social services.

RNID has been working hard to change GPs' attitudes. It has produced a guide for doctors and surgery staff to help ensure they communicate more effectively with their deaf and hard of hearing patients.

What happens in a hearing test

The hearing test (also called an audiometric test) is usually done at the ear, nose and throat (ENT) clinic or the hearing aid centre. The audiologist asks the person to put on a pair of headphones, and listen to a series of bleeps. They are asked to press a button every time they hear a bleep. The bleeps get quieter until the person can no longer hear them. Then they get louder again, by smaller steps, to find the precise point at which the person does begin to hear. The audiologist may also want to test at what level the sound is so loud that it becomes uncomfortable.

The audiogram

The audiologist will do the test at a number of different frequencies or pitches, to see whether high sounds or low sounds are most affected. All the results are plotted on a chart called an **audiogram**, rather like a graph. The amplitude or volume of the sound is measured in decibels (dBHL stands for decibel hearing level). The pitch or frequency of the sound is measured in hertz (Hz). A man's voice talking might be about 30 to 60 decibels containing frequencies in the range 100 to 8,000 hertz. A telephone ringing might be about 70 decibels at 2,000 to 4,000 hertz. A lorry engine revving might be 120 decibels and is about 125 hertz.

A point is marked on the audiogram for the softest sound the person can hear at each frequency. This is done for both ears, with the better ear usually being tested first. (The left ear is marked with an X and the right ear with an O.) By looking at the audiogram, the audiologist can work out the level of hearing loss in each ear, and the frequencies that are affected.

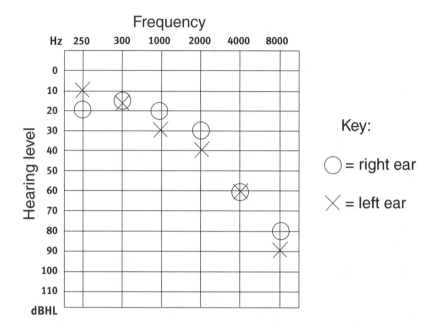

This audiogram shows a hearing loss for an older person with age-related deafness. This person has a high frequency hearing loss but has normal hearing in the low frequencies. (Diagram reproduced from RNID *All about hearing aids*.)

What kind of hearing loss?

To find out whether the hearing loss is caused by an obstruction stopping the sound getting through the ear canal (conductive loss) or to damage in the inner ear (sensorineural loss) the audiologist carries out another test. A small vibrator pad is pressed against the bone at the back of the ear, and this conducts sound through the bone of the skull, rather than through the ear canal.

When the sounds are presented, vibrations travel around the skull and can be heard in both ears at once. To test the bone conduction hearing of each ear separately, the audiologist may ask the person to wear headphones, and play a rushing sound through the headphones while presenting a sound through the vibrating pad.

11

If someone can hear better through bone conduction than air conduction, they have a conductive hearing loss. If their hearing is the same through bone conduction or through earphones, their hearing loss is sensorineural. (There is more about different kinds of hearing loss in Chapter 2.)

Measuring speech hearing loss

The tests above show how well a person can hear pure tones. But most sounds we hear in real life are made up of lots of different tones at different frequencies. Human speech, the most important sound for most of us, is an example of this.

The vowel sounds are low frequency sounds and consonants are higher frequency sounds. Most hearing loss through ageing occurs in the higher frequencies first, so sometimes the audiologist may want to test how the person hears and understands speech.

This is done by reading or playing a tape of a list of words, and asking the person to say or write the word, or touch the word on a screen. This is called **speech audiometry**. It is often only done if someone is being fitted for a hearing aid, or if the audiologist or ENT (ear, nose and throat) surgeon thinks there may be some damage to the inner ear or the hearing nerve itself.

For more *i*nformation

❶ The RNID Helpline (details on page 142).

❶ *It's time for a hearing test.* A report on hearing tests, ear health and public attitudes published by RNID, available at a cost of £4 from the address on page 142.

❶ *It's time to test your hearing* and *Top ten tips for people with a hearing loss*, leaflets available free from RNID (address on page 142).

❶ Contact Hearing Concern at the address on page 140.

2 Understanding hearing loss

Our ears are such delicate and wondrous organs, it is hardly surprising things go wrong from time to time. Around one in seven people are deaf or have a hearing loss, and the older we get, the more likely we are to be affected. More than half of people aged over 60 have some degree of hearing loss, and for many, the effect is very disabling, cutting them off from family and friends.

Growing older is the main cause of hearing loss, but it is by no means the only cause. Understanding the reason for the problem can help someone decide how best to deal with it. This chapter explains how the ear works, and describes some different kinds of hearing loss, including those affecting older people.

Pauline

'My mother went completely deaf on her 53rd birthday. She had been going deaf since her teens. It got gradually worse, and it seemed to get markedly worse after the birth of each child. She had had quite a few operations, and tried many different kinds of hearing aids. Just before she went completely deaf, she had been told she would not be able to have another operation, as it might affect her balance as well as her hearing.

'She'd started going to lipreading classes, and she thought she was prepared for the deafness, but nothing can prepare you for it. She woke up that morning and there was nothing there at all. She said the difference between going deaf and being completely deaf was terrible – no background noise, nothing.

'To a hearing person, the sound of silence can be lovely – but that's what it is – it's a sound. You could never begin to realise the difference between being hard of hearing and being completely deaf.'

Some facts and figures

There are about 8.7 million people in the UK who are either deaf or hard of hearing; that is one in seven of the population. When we look at the adult population, the figure is even higher. One in five adults have a hearing loss, but more than half of people aged over 60 have a hearing loss, and among people over 80, more than nine out of ten are either deaf or hard of hearing.

Talking about hearing loss

So what do we mean when we talk about **deafness** and **hearing loss**? Hearing loss is a broad term which can cover the whole range of hearing disability, from someone who is **profoundly deaf**, with no hearing at all, to someone who is slightly **hard of hearing**, and can understand so long as we speak clearly. **Hearing impaired**, usually used in educational or medical settings, is another broad term which can mean anything between these two extremes. When we say someone is **deaf** it usually implies that their hearing is severely impaired, although they may not be profoundly deaf.

Most professionals who work with deaf people distinguish between **pre-lingual deafness**, where someone was born deaf or became deaf before they learnt to talk, and **post-lingual deafness**, when someone has lost their hearing after they have learnt speech. This is an important distinction, because people who are pre-lingually deaf may have learnt sign language as their first language, and have learnt to speak only afterwards. Post-lingually deaf people, on the other hand, will have learnt to speak as children, and so English or another spoken language will be their first language. People who suddenly became deaf as adults are sometimes described as **deafened**.

Degrees of hearing loss

There are different degrees of hearing loss. We say that someone has a **mild** hearing loss if the quietest sounds they can hear are on average 25 to 40 decibels. That is about the sound level in a quiet sitting room. People with mild hearing loss can usually use a telephone and can follow a conversation, but they may find it helpful to lipread as well, especially if there is a lot of background noise. About 28 per cent of people aged from 61 to 80 and 18 per cent of people aged 81 or over have a mild hearing loss.

Madge

'I had mastoid operations on both ears when I was about 16. That was before the days of antibiotics. One surgeon said I would be totally deaf afterwards, so my parents took me to someone else, who saved my hearing. But a few years later I had to have another operation and my hearing started deteriorating again in that ear. However, my other ear was still satisfactory, or so I thought. But when an ENT specialist tested my ears, he said I ought to have a hearing aid.'

Someone has a **moderate** hearing loss if the quietest sounds they can hear are between 40 to 70 decibels. An ordinary spoken conversation is about 60 decibels, so someone with a moderate hearing loss will probably find it helpful to use a hearing aid. They should be able to use a telephone with an amplifier. About 16 per cent of people aged from 61 to 80, and 58 per cent of people aged 81 and over have a moderate hearing loss.

Severe deafness is when the quietest sounds someone can hear are between 70 to 95 decibels. The sound of someone shouting nearby is about 80 decibels. So even with a hearing aid, someone who is severely deaf will need to rely on lipreading to follow a conversation, and will need to use a textphone or videophone. Severe deafness is relatively uncommon. Fewer than 2 per cent of people aged 61 to 80 are severely deaf, and about 13 per cent of people aged 81 and over are severely deaf.

A **profoundly deaf** person is described as someone who can only hear sounds of 95 decibels or more. A pneumatic drill nearby makes a sound of 110 decibels. Some profoundly deaf people can use a hearing aid, but others rely on lipreading. If they have been deaf from an early age, they will probably use sign language. They will need a textphone or videophone.

How the ear works

The ear is an amazingly fine and complex organ, which collects sound waves from the environment, converts them into electrical signals, and sends them to the brain. It has three sections:

The outer ear

The part of the ear that sticks out at the side of your head is called the outer ear. It consists of the *pinna*, the part we can see, and the *external auditory canal* that leads down into the part of the ear which is inside the head. At the end of the auditory canal is the *eardrum*, sometimes called the *tympanic membrane*. Sounds travel down the auditory canal, and vibrate on the eardrum.

The middle ear

Beyond the eardrum is the middle ear. This is a cavity filled with air, and connected by the *eustachian tube* to the back of the

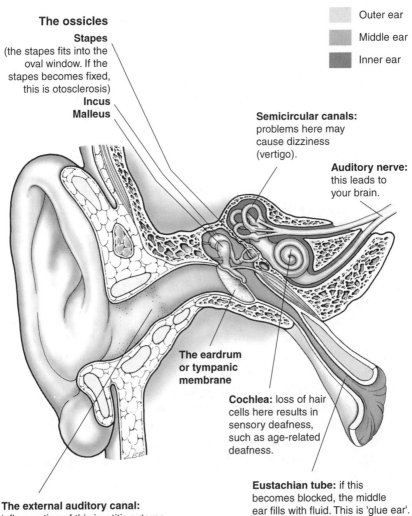

The ossicles
Stapes
(the stapes fits into the
oval window. If the
stapes becomes fixed,
this is otosclerosis)
Incus
Malleus

Outer ear
Middle ear
Inner ear

Semicircular canals:
problems here may
cause dizziness
(vertigo).

Auditory nerve:
this leads to
your brain.

**The eardrum
or tympanic
membrane**

Cochlea: loss of hair
cells here results in
sensory deafness,
such as age-related
deafness.

Eustachian tube: if this
becomes blocked, the middle
ear fills with fluid. This is 'glue ear'.

The external auditory canal:
inflammation of this is *otitis externa*.
Eczema or excessive wax may need treatment.
Blockages caused by excess wax may also occur here.

Diagram of the ear
(Source: RNID/Gillian Lee Illustrations)

17

nose and throat. Stretching across this cavity is a chain of three tiny bones called *ossicles*, which conduct the sound from the eardrum to the inner ear. The three ossicles are called the *incus*, the *malleus* and the *stapes*. The malleus, which is attached to the eardrum, acts like a little hammer, vibrating on the incus, which vibrates against the stapes. The stapes then pushes like a little piston against a membrane stretched across the *oval window*. The oval window links the middle ear to the inner ear.

The inner ear

The inner ear is the part that conducts messages to the brain. Inside the inner ear is the *cochlea*, a spiral coiled tube rather like a shell, which has two chambers filled with fluid. The outer chamber starts at the *oval window*, goes right round the cochlea, then curls back to the *round window*. When the stapes vibrates against the oval window, the sound is conducted along the fluid in the outer chamber of the cochlea.

The sound waves then travel along this fluid, moving tiny hairs in the central chamber of the cochlea. This is called the *Organ of Corti*. It contains about 17,000 small hair cells, and these are connected to the *auditory nerve*, which links the cochlea to the brain. The auditory nerve, which is also called the nerve of hearing, picks up the sound waves from the hair cells, and converts them into tiny electrical signals, which it sends to the brain. Different hair cells pick up different frequencies of sound. High frequency sounds are picked up by the hairs in one part of the cochlea spiral, low frequency sounds are picked up in another part. The brain interprets them as different sounds – voices, music, traffic.

Embedded in the bone of the inner ear, next to the cochlea, are the *semicircular canals*. These are not part of the hearing system, they are used for balance. Like the cochlea, they have thousands of tiny hair cells, and are filled with fluid. When you move your head, the fluid in the canals moves, and the hair cells pick up the movement and send messages to your brain about which way your head is moving.

Hearing loss in older people

We all tend to lose our hearing as we grow older, due to years of wear and tear on the tiny hair cells in the cochlea. This is the most common cause of deafness in the population, but few people know its medical name. **Presbyacusis** is the name of the natural loss of hearing that comes with ageing. Often the hair cells in the cochlea that pick up high frequency sounds are the first to go, so that although you can hear people talking, you lose the consonants, and it sounds as though everyone is mumbling.

Most people who develop presbyacusis rely increasingly on lip-reading – sometimes without even being aware that they are doing so. A hearing aid can be very helpful too, but it should be carefully set, so that it amplifies in those frequencies that are worst affected.

Other common hearing problems

With so many delicate parts, the ear is very vulnerable to damage which can lead to deafness. If the sound waves cannot pass through the outer or middle ear, because of blockage, accident or infection, this is called **conductive deafness**. If the deafness is caused by damage to the cochlea or the auditory nerve it is called **sensorineural deafness**.

Problems of the outer ear

The outer ear, the part you can see, is vulnerable to infections, injury and blockages. Some common problems are:

Ear wax is secreted in the ear to keep it clean, but it can build up, causing loss of hearing. It is best to see the doctor or practice nurse, and ask them about removing the wax from the ears. It is very dangerous to try to remove the ear wax yourself by poking cotton buds or anything else into the ear.

Otitis is an inflammation of the skin inside the ear canal. *Otitis externa* is when the external auditory canal becomes inflamed, usually as a result of a scratch or infection. The ear can become sore and weep a watery discharge. If this happens, a doctor will probably prescribe ear drops and maybe antibiotics as well.

Perforated eardrums may be caused by an explosion, sudden loud noise, diving, poking something sharp into the ear, using over-heated olive oil, or other accidental injuries. The result is always sudden deafness. Occasionally, the perforation heals up on its own, or can be repaired with a skin-graft operation called a *myringoplasty*.

Problems of the middle ear

Glue ear, or *otitis media*, is very common in young children. It happens when the eustachian tube is blocked and air cannot get into the middle ear cavity, which fills up with a thick sticky fluid instead. This stops the eardrum from vibrating, resulting in loss of hearing. Glue ear usually clears up on its own and does not cause permanent hearing loss. However, children with glue ear can fall behind in their speech and learning, so they may be offered an operation called a *myringotomy*, in which a small temporary ventilation tube called a grommet is inserted into the eardrum allowing air to get into the middle ear, so the sticky fluid can dry up.

Chronic infection of the middle ear used to be a common cause of hearing loss, but is now unusual, thanks to modern antibiotics. However, dead skin can build up behind the eardrum as a result of infection, and may need to be removed through a mastoid operation before it permanently damages the hearing.

Otosclerosis is when the stapes, one of the ossicles, becomes enlarged and rigid as a result of bone overgrowth. Sound vibrations cannot pass through it and the person becomes progressively more deaf. This happens more commonly to women than men, and may start when they are in their 30s. Heredity is thought to play a part. An operation called a *stapedectomy* can often help by replacing the stapes with a tiny piston which transmits sound to the inner ear. A *stapedotomy* removes a small part of the stapes and replaces it with a pinhead-sized prosthesis.

Problems of the inner ear

When damage occurs in the inner ear, the result is **sensorineural deafness**, meaning that the senses cannot send messages to the brain. The most common form of deafness in older people, **presbyacusis** (see above), results from natural wear and tear to the tiny hair cells in the cochlea. However, these hair cells can also be damaged in other ways:

- If the mother has rubella (German measles) while she is pregnant the baby may be born with damaged hearing.
- A baby's ears can be damaged in labour, or if the baby is born prematurely.
- Diseases such as mumps and meningitis can cause deafness.
- Some drugs, such as aspirin or antibiotics called streptomycin and gentamicin can very rarely cause deafness.
- Through working for a long time in a noisy environment.
- Through a serious head injury resulting in skull fracture.

For more *i*nformation

ⓘ RNID booklets: *How your ears work; Deaf and hard of hearing people; Age-related hearing loss* and *Common ear problems*, all available free from the RNID Helpline (details on page 142).

3 Improving communication

Someone who has become deaf gradually over a period of time will probably have worked out their own best way of communicating. They will have got used to looking carefully as well as listening. They may have learnt to read clues from facial expression, gestures and body language, without even being aware of it. They will know they can follow a conversation better if they turn off the television or radio. In fact they may have become so good at 'managing' communication that they aren't aware they have a hearing loss.

If the person you care for only has a mild hearing loss, they may be able to communicate without a hearing aid in many situations. Most people who do use a hearing aid also depend on lipreading and reading body language. Whichever way the person you care for communicates, there is much they – and you – can do to make it easier.

Freda

'If you want to communicate with someone with a hearing loss, my advice is, be patient with them. Find out how you can help, but first accept what has happened and be supportive. A sense of humour helps. Very many funny situations will arise. Do be interested. A problem shared is a problem halved.'

Planning what you say

By thinking carefully about what you say and how you say it, you can make it much easier for someone with hearing loss to understand you.

Try to spend a few seconds planning what you are going to say before you start to talk. These hints will make it easier for someone who lipreads to follow what you are saying:

- Get the person's attention, and make sure they are watching you before you start to speak.
- Indicate that you are introducing a new topic of conversation, so that the person you are talking with knows what words to listen and look out for. This will make it easier to predict what might be coming next.
- Put 'key words' near the beginning, then repeat them from time to time. That way, the other person will know that you're still on the same topic – or they will know if the topic has changed.
- Use simple grammar with one main idea to each sentence. For example: 'I saw Mary today. She's got new job. She's working in a shoe shop.' This is easier to follow than: 'By the way, have you heard about Mary's new job in the shoe shop? I bumped into her today and she was telling me all about it.'
- If you are asked to repeat something, try to say it in a different, simpler way.
- Be aware that some words are easier to lipread than others. Words where the sound is made by the tongue and lips are easier to lipread than words where the sound is made in the throat.
- Check from time to time that the other person is following the conversation, by asking an open question – that is, a question that doesn't take a yes or no answer. For example, if you ask, 'Do you like Mary's new boyfriend?' someone may nod or say yes even if they haven't a clue what you're talking about. But if you ask, 'What do you think of Mary's boyfriend?' the person will only be able to reply if they have understood. That way, you will know whether they are following the conversation.

23

■ Don't assume that just because someone is nodding and saying 'yes' they are following what you're saying. They may nod and say 'yes' just to encourage you to keep on speaking in the hope that they will pick up a clue to the conversation sooner or later.

Annie

'We pretend we're not deaf, and say "Yes" and "No" and hope for the best. You feel a nuisance if you keep asking people to repeat things. You lipread a bit. You can tell someone's asked a question, so you say "Yes" or "No". Then you can tell from the look on somebody's face whether you said the right thing.'

Judith

'The more you don't get it, the more your stress level goes up, and the less you get it.'

Cutting down background noise

Background noise can make it much harder to follow a conversation, even for people without hearing difficulties, so it is especially important to cut out unwanted noise when you're talking with someone who has hearing loss. TV and radio, music, traffic noise, voices, clatter of cutlery, footsteps, alarms and sirens are just a few of the sounds which surround us in our everyday lives. Most of us learn to ignore them. But for someone with hearing loss, it is harder to distinguish between the unwanted background noise and the sound of the voice or voices they *do* want to hear.

Here are some helpful tips for cutting down on background noise:

- Choose a quiet place. If you are in a noisy environment, try to find a quiet corner.
- Sit or stand quite close to the person – about three feet away – but don't shout.
- Choose a place with good acoustics. Carpets and soft furnishings help muffle footsteps and clatter, and reduce echoing. Indoors is better than outdoors.
- Turn off the television, radio or music before you start to talk.

Harry

'One thing that annoys me on the radio – they will talk over the music. I find it hard to listen to music, because it all sounds flat to me. Joan, my wife, loves music, but when she talks to me she turns it off.'

Note **Remember a hearing aid may amplify unwanted background noise as well as your conversation.**

Making lipreading easier

We all find it easier to follow what someone is saying if we follow their lip movements, and this applies even more to someone who has a hearing loss. If you have ever tried to watch a film that has been dubbed from a foreign language, you will know how important lip movements are in helping us to understand what someone is saying. Someone who uses a hearing aid will find lipreading very helpful.

When you talk to someone who is using lipreading to understand you, remember:

- Make sure they can see your face, and that they are looking at you when you start to speak.
- Make sure you are facing towards them when you speak.

- Don't stand in front of a window or light so that your face is in the shadow.
- Try to be on the same level as the other person, so that they're not looking up or down at you.
- Moustaches, beards, dangly earrings, big hats all make it harder to see your face.
- Keep your hands away from your face. Don't talk and eat or drink at the same time.
- Speak slowly, but not too slowly.
- Don't exaggerate your lip movements – this will only confuse people.
- Use natural facial expressions and move your head naturally, but don't move about too much as you talk.
- Don't shout, as this will distort both your voice and your facial expression.

Arnold

'The most important thing, when you are talking to someone who is deaf, is to move your lips. Some people hardly move their mouth when they talk, and it's even worse if they've got a moustache. I can follow people on TV by lipreading if I can see their face, but some of them are always moving their heads around or talking with their back turned.'

Lipreading is not easy. A lot of the sounds have the same lip movement, for example *Sh*, *Ch* and *J*. Words such as *bat*, *mat* and *pat* all look the same. So you may have to be patient, and try to find different ways of saying things.

Lipreading requires tremendous concentration and mental effort, as the person has to rapidly work out which of two or three possible words with the same lip-shape make most sense in the context of what you are saying. Most people who lipread can only keep it up for a certain amount of time, and then mentally switch off to give themselves a rest.

Chris

'I have two hearing aids, but I still depend on lipreading to support my hearing. I can use fingerspelling or sign language too if necessary. Lipreading is part of my life. It's absolutely essential. It bothers me when people do things which make it harder to lipread, such as covering their mouth with their hands, or speaking with their head down.'

Zia

'My Grandad is a bit deaf now, but he can still follow what people are saying by lipreading in his own language. He finds it much harder when people are speaking in English, even though he has lived in this country for 32 years.'

Harry

'If you ask some people to repeat what they said, they think, "Oh, he's deaf", so they shout at you. That doesn't help at all.'

Phyllis

'I have two hearing aids, but I still find it difficult to hear people. I have to be close to them, and face to face. It's better if you face the light, and don't move your head about when you talk.'

Note **Remember, even if someone is using a hearing aid, they will probably still need to lipread.**

Lipreading classes

Chris

'The psychological problems of hearing loss may be worse than the physical ones. The physical problems can often be overcome with a good hearing aid, but to get over the psychological problems is much harder. This is why lipreading classes can help. You need to be with other people like you in a safe environment. You need people who will laugh with you, not at you, so you can face the fact that you make mistakes.'

Many people who go deaf later in life learn to lipread more efficiently by going to special classes. These are usually run by the local college, community centre or the social services department. Your social services department should be able to give you details of classes in your area, or you could ring the college directly.

We all lipread to some extent, but going to classes can really speed up the learning process, by showing the link between sounds and lip movements in a systematic way. There are also plenty of opportunities for practice without the risk of embarrassment.

Another big advantage of lipreading classes is that they're a good way of meeting other people with hearing loss. Classes are fun, and can be quite a social focus. Isolation is a major problem for many people with hearing loss, so this is an important point to consider if you want to encourage the person you care for to go to lipreading classes.

Harry

'When I first went deaf I felt terribly isolated. I lost all my confidence. I found myself opting out of things. Going to lipreading classes gave me back my confidence. Now I realise there's a lot of people like me.'

Chris

'I always say to people, go to lipreading classes now, before you think you need it, and while you've still got your confidence, before your family start getting at you. Don't ignore the warning signs like having the TV turned up too loud or getting irritated with people because you think they're mumbling. As soon as you have a mild hearing impairment, go and learn the basics. You need the confidence just to look at people before you can even begin to lipread. You won't lose the basics, and you can build up gradually.'

Sign language

Many people who have been deaf from birth, or have become deaf early in life, learn to communicate through sign language. British Sign Language (BSL) is used by about 50,000 people in Britain. For some, it is the first language they learn; others learn it at school or when they meet other sign language users. Like any language, it has its own grammar, which is different to English grammar, and enables the same rich and expressive communication. And like any language, it has its own community of users, the Deaf Community in Britain. If someone from the Deaf Community wants to communicate with people who do not know sign language, they may need to use an interpreter.

At one time it was thought that learning sign language would make learning spoken language more difficult, and deaf people were actively encouraged to learn to speak instead. Now it is generally recognised that sign language, by breaking down isolation and allowing deaf people to communicate freely, is a great benefit.

Pauline

'Mother went gradually deaf as we were growing up, so without realising it, we sort of developed our own sign language within the family. Then when she lost her hearing completely, we went and learnt sign language with her. What we found was that a lot of the signs we'd used in the family were the same as the "official" BSL signs – a lot of it's common sense, really.'

So should the person you care for be encouraged to learn sign language? That depends very much on their age and their degree of hearing loss.

If someone's hearing loss is so profound that they cannot use a hearing aid at all, then sign language may be the best or only way that they can communicate. However, this will only allow them to communicate with other people who have learned sign language, and who are part of the Deaf Community.

Most people who become deaf later in life have already put down their family and social roots among people who can hear. Losing all one's familiar social contacts is as upsetting as losing one's hearing. So if they can manage to communicate with the use of a hearing aid and lipreading they usually choose this.

Judith

'I lipread and lip-speak, and now I have learnt to sign. It took me three years. It's a very beautiful, very expressive language. It uses the whole body from the waist up. However, problems can arise because deaf people were prevented from signing for so long. Now they have developed their own sign language community, but hard of hearing people can feel left out.'

> ### Doreen
>
> 'I can speak several languages, so I decided to try sign language. It came as a surprise to learn that sign language has dialects, just like other languages. For example, even Sheffield and Derby have different signs to Chesterfield for some words.'

I hate it when ...

People with a hearing loss often say how irritated they get when people ignore their needs, and put all the onus on the hard of hearing person, when just a little bit of thought would make communication so much easier. Here are some pet hates:

- People talking and eating at the same time.
- People talking and chewing gum at the same time.
- People talking and writing (looking down) at the same time – doctors are especially criticised for this.
- People talking and moving their head at the same time.
- People talking and smoking at the same time.
- People talking from another room, or from upstairs.
- People wearing dark glasses – facial expression provides important clues to speech.
- Being made fun of when asking someone to repeat something.
- Asking someone to repeat something and being told, 'Oh, it doesn't matter'.

Other ways of communicating

Some people use a mixture of speech and signing. This is called **Sign Supported English (SSE)** and is more often used by people who lost their hearing after they learned to speak, but who are part of a network of deaf people.

Most people with hearing loss get used to carrying a **notepad and pen** around with them. However, these are not always convenient to use.

Fingerspelling is a way of making the shapes of letters with your fingers. It's not the same as sign language, where every sign stands for a whole word or phrase. With fingerspelling you have to show every letter, so it's rather slow. But it's useful for communicating names and difficult or unusual words if no paper and pen are handy. Fingerspelling is often used by people who lipread to understand difficult or unfamiliar words. It is also used by people who use sign language for names when there is no specific sign.

Help with communication

There will be situations in which it's important to make sure that the person you care for understands what is said, and can make themselves understood, for example at the doctor's, or in hospital.

If the person knows sign language, then a **sign language interpreter** may be able to help.

People who rely on lipreading may find it helpful to have a **lipspeaker**, that is someone who repeats the speaker's message very clearly, but without using their voice so that it is clear to lipread.

In a situation where a lot of information needs to be given, then someone who relies on lipreading or on watching a sign language interpreter, may need a **notetaker** as well.

The lighter side of life

Hearing loss is a serious condition, but people who have accepted their hearing loss and no longer feel ashamed of it, can share a joke about some of the funny or embarrassing situations they have found themselves in.

Pauline

'Mum was talking to a woman at the bus stop. The woman was smiling as she talked – well it was more a sort of embarrassed grin because she felt awkward. Mum couldn't hear what she was saying, so she just responded to what she thought was the other woman's smile, smiling back and saying, "Oh, lovely! That's lovely!" When the woman walked away, I said, "Mum, why were you saying, "Oh, lovely", when that woman was telling you how her husband died?"'

Ann Mawkes

'When I first became deaf, I got into the habit of saying, "Yes" when I couldn't hear what people said to me. At that time our house was up for sale. A prospective buyer came to look around while it was pouring with rain. My husband told me she'd said "Oh, I must look a sight." To which I had said, "Yes". So that taught me a lesson, and now I know it is best to own up right away to deafness.'*

Notice on the front door of a house in Wellington, New Zealand:

'To Postman – I'm out, but dog is in. Ring bell and he will bark, setting off dog next door. His master is hard of hearing but when he sees his dog barking, he'll come to the door. Leave letters with him!'*

*Reprinted with kind permission from: *Read My Lips, Hear My Hands: Stories, anecdotes and verse written by members of the Deaf and Hard of Hearing Community of Sheffield.*

For more *i*nformation

ⓘ Hearing Concern Helpline: 01245 344600.

ⓘ *Lipreading: A guide for beginners* by John Chaloner Woods, published by RNID (address on page 142).

ⓘ *No Need to Shout* published by ITV Books in Association with Tyne Tees Television.

ⓘ *Learning British Sign Language* factsheet from RNID.

ⓘ *Deaf Awareness Curriculum* available from the Council for the Advancement of Communication with Deaf People (address on page 138).

ⓘ *Read My Lips, Hear My Hands: Stories, anecdotes and verse written by members of the Deaf and Hard of Hearing Community of Sheffield.* Available from the Deaf Advisory Service, Sheffield. Tel: 0114 2780410.

ⓘ *Start to Sign* by Richard Magill and Anne Hodgson, published by RNID.

ⓘ *To hear or not to hear* and *I'm only deaf*: videos on dealing with an acquired hearing loss, available from The Forest Bookshop which has a mail order catalogue of books, videos and CD-ROMs about deafness and deaf issues (address on page 140).

4 Using a hearing aid

Using a hearing aid can transform the life of someone with hearing loss, yet only about half of the four million people in this country who could benefit actually wear one. Getting the right hearing aid is important, but learning how to use it correctly is essential too. There are often teething troubles when a new hearing aid is fitted, and the benefits of wearing it do not always outweigh the difficulties at first. But it really pays to persevere. You may need to give plenty of help and encouragement until the person gets used to their new aid and learns how to make the most of it.

Rene

'I had one of the first hearing aids that ever came out. In those days they gave everybody the same one, regardless of need. It was a huge thing – part of it on the front and part of it down the side, with a big wire that went up the back. It's in a museum now. But it changed my life.'

Madge

'My hearing aid is digital. It's small, but the sound is very clear, and it's been set by computer to match my hearing loss, so it just boosts the range of sounds I find hardest to hear.'

Feelings about hearing aids

Hearing aids can make an enormous difference. So why do so many people put off getting one? And why, having got one, do so many people use it for a couple of weeks then just put it in a drawer and never get it out again?

Wearing a hearing aid means admitting in public that one has a hearing problem. That can be hard to do, especially as there can be a stigma attached to hearing loss.

Albert

'It takes a while to pluck up the courage to get assessed. A lot of people who have hearing aids don't wear them out of embarrassment. They don't want everybody to know they're deaf.'

Sometimes there are practical reasons why the hearing aid is put away and forgotten about. The person you care for may be partially sighted or have arthritis or another illness or disability which makes it difficult for them to master their hearing aid.

Peter

'I thought having a hearing aid would change my life, but when I got it home, it was so fiddly I found it hard to use. I have bad arthritis in my hands. I can't manage the controls. I keep thinking that one day I'll get it out again. Maybe if my hearing gets really bad I'll have another go.'

If someone has been deaf for a while, the shock of suddenly re-entering the hearing world may be too much for them.

Chris

'At first when I went out, I thought, "How can people put up with it – the background noise, the traffic?" Then someone told me, "They don't – they just switch it off in those situations."'

Learning how to manage the hearing aid so as to minimise background noise and discomfort is important. People who have overcome those initial obstacles say they wouldn't be without their hearing aid.

Rene

'When we got married my husband bought me an expensive hearing aid that was fixed onto my spectacles. It cost £80, and his wage was £5 a week. I now have two modern high-powered hearing aids. I'm most pleased with them. They're the first thing I put on after my bath in the mornings and the last thing I take off at night. I've never been tempted to put them in a drawer. The best thing is, with them on I'm in a world that's alive.'

Don't put it off

If the person you care for has not had a hearing test, encourage them to do it as soon as possible. There are two reasons for this.

Firstly, there is plenty of evidence to show that the younger a person is when they start with their hearing aid, the more likely they are to make a success of using it, and to get the maximum benefit from it.

Secondly, they are likely to encounter delays and queues in getting their hearing tested on the NHS, so the sooner they get on the waiting list the better.

Where to go for help

The GP

The first port of call for any hearing problem is the family doctor (also called the GP or general practitioner). The GP will make an initial assessment and make sure there is not some straightforward problem such as an infection or earwax that can easily be cleared up in the surgery. Some GPs tend to think of hearing loss as a 'normal' part of the ageing process, so if the hearing loss is not severe, they may not want to refer the person to the hospital at all, and they may need to be persuaded. If the GP decides the person needs further tests, he or she may refer them to the specialist in the local ENT (ear, nose and throat) department at your local hospital. There may be quite a long waiting list for the first appointment to see the consultant.

The GP may be able to refer someone directly to the hearing aid clinic within the hospital audiology department, without having to wait to see an ENT specialist. This usually applies only to people over 60, and depends on the policy of your local health trust.

A few GPs' surgeries and health centres run audiology clinics in their own centres where someone can have their hearing tested without going to hospital.

Freda

'My hearing loss was very gradual. I first became aware of it when answering the phone at work. It wasn't until after I retired that I approached my doctor, and it took another year to convince her before she made an appointment for me to see the ear, nose and throat specialist.'

The hospital audiology department

If the person you care for goes through an ENT (ear, nose and throat) department, the ENT consultant will examine both ears and find out about the patient's medical history. The patient will then see the audiologist for a hearing test (audiogram). The audiogram will show the degree of hearing loss, and will also show the frequencies that are most affected and whether the loss is conductive or sensorineural. In age-related hearing loss, it is usually the higher frequencies which are affected first, but as the hearing loss gets worse, other frequencies are affected too. (There is more about the audiogram on pages 10–11.)

The audiogram will show how much hearing loss has occurred, and whether a hearing aid would help. If a hearing aid is needed, the audiologist will take an impression of the ear by filling the ear with impression material that takes a few minutes to set. This is used to make an earmould that exactly fits inside the ear. It is important to get a good fit, so that sound from the hearing aid does not leak out and cause feedback (an annoying whistling noise). It may take a few weeks for the mould to be made.

When it is ready, the person needs to make another appointment to have the hearing aid fitted, and to learn how to use it and look after it.

Some audiology departments also have a **hearing therapist** who can advise about all aspects of hearing loss, and help with other ways of improving communication. In other departments, help and support are given by the audiologist.

You may find it helpful to go along with the person you care for to these appointments, so you can make sure that you both understand how the hearing aid works, and learn some basic 'troubleshooting' hints. You will also be able to get to know the staff in the audiology department, in case you need to contact them in future.

Rene

'I had my first hearing aid fitted just after the war. We had the repairs done in a small pokey room at the top of a flight of stairs on a landing at the end of the men's geriatric ward. I remember the old men used to wander around in various forms of dress and undress, trousers undone or in some cases down. The repairs were carried out by the hospital electrician. Now we have a most efficiently-run audiology department, where care is second to none. The hearing therapist is always on hand to listen and help, gives lipreading lessons, and is most kind.'

As a person with hearing loss grows older, their hearing will probably continue to deteriorate, so you will most likely develop an ongoing relationship with the staff in the audiology department.

How the hearing aid works

A hearing aid has three parts: a **microphone**, which picks up the sounds; an **amplifier**, which makes the sounds louder; and an **earphone**, which transmits the amplified sound into the ear. It is powered by a tiny battery.

When the hearing aid is switched on, the microphone detects sounds within its range, and sends them to the amplifier. The amplifier boosts the volume of the sound according to how high the setting is. This is then transmitted right into the ear via the earphone.

It is important to understand how the hearing aid works, because then you can understand what it can and cannot do. A hearing aid cannot cure deafness or give back normal hearing. What it can do is magnify the sound that is already there, so that someone who has lost some of their hearing will be able to hear better.

A hearing aid is not as sophisticated as an ear. Most do not distinguish between different kinds of sounds. The microphone of the hearing aid picks up **all** the sound in the environment – background noise, traffic, the voices of all people talking in the room, not just the one you want to listen to. It amplifies **all** these sounds and sends them to the ear. This is why people often have difficulties when they first start using a hearing aid.

Harry

'When you first get a hearing aid, it's a bit like those railway announcers used to be. It's very loud, but you can't always make out what they're saying.'

Zia

'My Grandad uses his hearing aid when he goes out, but when it's something really important he usually takes me or my brother with him because he's worried he might miss something.'

Different types of hearing aid

All hearing aids do the same job – of helping people to hear better – but may not work in the same way. They do not look the same, they have different controls and settings and are worn differently. The most common kind of hearing aids are behind-the-ear (BTE) models and in-the-ear (ITE) models, and one of these will suit most people. BTE models are the sort usually prescribed on the National Health Service. ITE models are usually available only privately, and they can be very expensive, but some people who wear them much prefer them. These and other less common solutions are described below.

Behind-the-ear (BTE) hearing aids

The main parts of the hearing aid, the microphone, amplifier and earphone, sit snugly behind the ear. A narrow tube connects the hearing aid to the earmould in the ear.

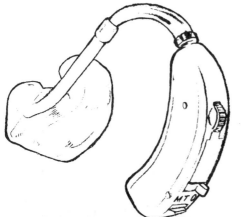

*Typical behind-the-ear aid
with earmould*

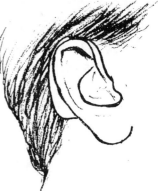

(Crown copyright material is
reproduced with the permission
of the Controller of Her
Majesty's Stationery Office.)

Wearing a behind-the-ear aid

These hearing aids are suitable for most people with mild, moderate, severe or profound hearing loss, and are available on the NHS. There are different models to choose from, depending on the amplification needed. The audiologist will recommend the best one based on the results of the hearing tests, and the hearing aid will be specially tuned to the person's needs.

Annie

'I'm 93, and I have an NHS BE34 model. Without it, I can't hear much. With it, I can hear too much. That says it all.'

In-the-ear (ITE) hearing aids

These are much smaller than the behind-the-ear models. The whole of the hearing aid – the microphone, amplifier and earphone – are all inside the earmould which sits in the ear, making it much less visible. The earmoulds can come in different colours, which can be matched to the person's skin tone. Some very small aids fit right inside the ear canal and are called in-the-canal (ITC) or completely-in-the-canal (CIC) hearing aids. They cannot be seen.

Although the ITE hearing aid is very small, it can be quite powerful. However, they are not suitable for everyone. People who have very narrow ears, or have a tendency towards ear infections, and people with severe or profound hearing loss will probably be advised to use a different kind of hearing aid. ITE hearing aids are expensive and most are bought privately. Modular ITE aids, which consist of a tiny hearing aid clipped to a custom-made earmould, are available on the NHS.

There are many different models of in-the-ear aid, but they are not suitable for everyone.

Ethel

'I've got two aids, one in each ear. I got them privately. I have very small ears, and I found the NHS behind-the-ear ones didn't fit very well. They kept on slipping. I have mainly high-tone deafness, so I can never hear birdsong, and I don't hear the telephone when it rings, but I'm not too bad with the lower sounds.'

Digital hearing aids

Digital hearing aids are fitted with a tiny computer chip that processes the sound in a different way, making it clearer and sharper as well as louder. Some digital aids can be worn in the ear, and there are behind-the-ear models.

Some can be programmed by a computer to amplify just those frequencies which have suffered most hearing loss. With most older

43

people, this is high-pitched sounds and consonants like 's', 'k', 't'. The latest digital aids adjust automatically to different sounds, and can distinguish the human voice from other background sounds.

These aids have not been generally available on the NHS, but they are now being introduced in some regions as part of a two-year pilot scheme, and it is hoped that they will soon become more widely available. Contact your local audiology department or RNID for more information. Meanwhile, they can still be bought privately, but the cost is likely to be up to £2,500.

Harry

'I had a digital aid on a five-week trial, and I must say, it was marvellous. The difference was, you just didn't get the background noise. The aid automatically tuned in to speech. I could hear when Joan spoke to me, even in the car. Even with the radio or tape on I could hear her voice. She plays the organ, and I've never liked to listen to it because it always sounded a bit flat. But with the digital aid, it sounded like music. We went to the theatre, an amateur show, and even though I was sitting five rows back, I could hear every word.

'The best thing is – it's fully automatic. It has different channels, and it automatically selects the right one for the sound conditions. You don't need a volume control or a T-switch. You don't have to fiddle with it. That's important, because as you get older your fingers aren't so nimble. I really wanted to keep it. Joan begged me to keep it. But at the end of the five weeks I sent it back. The trouble is, it was £1,500, and that's a lot of money for a pensioner.'

Body-worn aids

These are powerful aids which are larger than the others and are worn on the body. The main parts of the hearing aid – the microphone, amplifier and batteries – are housed in a special pack a little bigger than a matchbox, which is clipped to the clothes or carried in a pocket. A discreet lead connects the hearing aid to the earmould. They are more powerful aids and have bigger batteries. They are not used so much nowadays, as powerful behind-the-ear hearing aids have been designed, but they may still be the best choice for someone with severe or profound hearing loss.

Bone-conduction hearing aids

The skull-bone behind the ear conducts sound vibrations to the inner ear. A bone-conduction hearing aid makes use of this by pressing against the bone and amplifying these vibrations. A bone-conduction hearing aid is usually worn on a headset with a steel spring arch over the head. This is a bit more visible than other hearing aids, and some people find it uncomfortable to wear for a very long period of time. It can be useful for someone with con-ductive hearing loss who cannot wear an earmould in their ear, for example if their ear canal is infected or damaged. A bone-conduc-tion aid can also be fitted to the frame of a pair of spectacles.

Bone-anchored hearing aids

Bone-anchored hearing aids (BAHA) are similar to bone-conduc-tion hearing aids (above) except that they are anchored directly to the skull by a small titanium screw that is implanted behind the ear. The operation is straightforward, and can be carried out under local anaesthetic. After about three months, when the screw has settled and integrated into the bone, a little clip is fitted to it, and this little clip is used to anchor the hearing aid. The hearing aid is quite small and can be hidden under the hair. It can be taken on and off, but the screw and clip stay firmly in position. A BAHA may be a good solution for some people with conductive hearing loss.

Spectacle hearing aids

People who need spectacles and a hearing aid can sometimes combine the two by having a hearing aid fitted to one or both arms of the spectacles. This can be a neat solution, but it can cause difficulties as the aid cannot be separated from the spectacles. Many people use different spectacles for different situations, for example reading and driving. There could also be a problem if one or the other needs to be repaired.

CROS/BiCROS hearing aids

These can be helpful for people who have reasonably good hearing in one ear but have lost their hearing in the other, maybe as a result of an accident or injury. The CROS hearing aid feeds sound from the ear which has lost its hearing into the good ear. The BiCROS aid amplifies sounds from both sides and feeds them into the best ear (see page 135).

Cochlear implants

The tiny hair cells of the cochlea transmit sound waves to the auditory nerve (see page 17). If these hair cells are damaged or not working properly the sound does not reach the brain. This is an example of sensorineural hearing loss (see page 21). If the damage to the hair cells is very severe, the person will be severely or profoundly deaf. A cochlear implant is one of the few ways of providing some hearing to a person with a profound hearing loss. A microphone that looks like a behind-the-ear hearing aid picks up sounds, which are conducted to a speech processor. From there, fine wires conduct the sound to a tiny transmitter implanted surgically right inside the ear.

A cochlear implant may be considered suitable for children who have been born with this kind of sensorineural deafness, or become deaf very early in life. There is some controversy about whether such children should be fitted with implants, or encouraged to develop as members of the Deaf Community, communicating through sign language. Cochlear implants may be offered to older people, depending on the policy of the local Health Trust. A cochlear implant will not help if the auditory nerve itself is damaged.

Pauline

'My mother had been completely deaf for ten years, and was told there was no chance of her ever hearing again, when she heard about what was then a new operation – the cochlear implant. She was among the first people in the region to have the operation, and she had to keep a diary of her experience. It was switched on six weeks after the operation, and we were all there. You should have seen the look on her face.

'Really, it's just a glorified hearing aid that's mapped by computer. She has to go back regularly for mapping sessions. It's not given her her hearing back, but it has made her more aware of the hearing she has. Sometimes I go in and see her listening to the clock ticking, or rustling the newspapers and she says, "Listen – isn't it a wonderful sound?"'

Hearing aids with special features

Modern technology means that the newest hearing aids don't just amplify sound – they can also adapt and alter the sound that comes into the ear to make it easier and more comfortable to hear.

- **Tone control** means the hearing aid can be set to amplify lower or higher frequencies.
- **Automatic gain control** means that sounds are never amplified too much, making them uncomfortably loud. Very loud sound waves entering the aid or microphone are automatically compressed, in a way which does not distort them.
- **Peak clipping** is a similar feature – it means that when very loud sounds enter the microphone, the sound waves are clipped. Sometimes this gives a distorting effect.
- **Pre-programmed aids** have a number of different settings for different situations, for example talking face to face with one person, watching television, talking when there is a lot of background noise, T position (see below). These usually come with a remote control, so the person can switch discreetly from programme to programme without fiddling with their aid.

47

The T-switch

Most modern hearing aids have three settings: 'M', 'T' and 'O'. 'M', for microphone, means the hearing aid is switched on; 'T' stands for telecoil; 'O' is off.

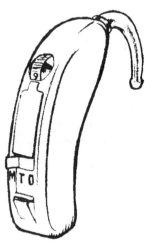

Most hearing aids can be switched into three positions: M (microphone – on), T (telecoil – loop) and O (off).

(Crown copyright material is reproduced with the permission of the Controller of Her Majesty's Stationery Office.)

When the hearing aid is switched to the T position, it means it is set to pick up sound not from the environment but from an induction loop or telecoil. Using a hearing aid switched to the T position means that only sound picked up by the loop is amplified, so confusing background noise is eliminated and the intended sounds are much clearer. Induction loops are used in many public buildings, and counters at banks, building societies, some shops, post office counters, railway ticket sales counters, and most public telephones. (For more about induction loops, see Chapters 5 and 7.)

Most behind-the-ear models, and many in-the-ear models, have a T-switch, but some very small hearing aids may be too small to have one. This is a question to ask the person fitting the hearing aid.

Making the most of hearing aids

Starting gradually

Whatever the type of hearing aid, it takes some time to learn how to use it to full effect. The longer someone has had a hearing loss, the longer it will take for them to get used to hearing again with an aid. The first time someone uses a hearing aid, the effect can be quite overwhelming. It is at this point that many people who have gone to great lengths to get their hearing aid, decide to put it in a drawer and leave it there.

For this reason, many hearing therapists or audiology technicians advise new hearing aid users to wear their aid for just half an hour every day at first, increasing this as they get more used to it. It's best to start indoors, where there is generally less background noise, and to gradually get used to the amplified sound. Encourage them to listen to everyday sounds with the hearing aid in, so they will recognise them and then gradually let them slip into the back of their mind, rather than being intensely aware of them.

Remember, a hearing aid can always be adjusted. Many users take them back for adjustment several times until they are happy with the fit and the level of the sound. Older people sometimes feel they don't want to be a nuisance, but it's more important to get the hearing aid right so it can be used daily, rather than putting up with one which isn't satisfactory and stays in the drawer.

Harry

'My hearing aid helps me a lot. The problem is, with it being more powerful, it picks up more background noise. At first everything was so loud, I took it back and asked them to adjust it to cut out the background noise. But I found I couldn't hear what people were saying, so I had to go back and ask them to turn it up again.'

Persevering

The person you care for may need plenty of encouragement to persevere through this difficult stage. Most people find it difficult to adjust to using a hearing aid. A positive attitude from their carers and family will help them feel less clumsy and stupid. You can help by making a point of talking to them and involving them in family activities while they are trying out their hearing aid, so that they can begin to appreciate the difference it can make to their lives. At the same time, discourage them from using their hearing aid outdoors or in noisy and public situations until they are quite confident about using it.

Ethel

'I can remember when I first had my hearing aid fitted. As soon as she put it in my ear, I could hear the clock ticking. That was marvellous. But I didn't like wearing it outside at first because of all the traffic noise. I turned it down, and got used to it gradually.'

Some experiences of hearing aids

Chris

'It took about 10 months to get my first hearing aid. However, when I got it I felt too embarrassed to put it in, and it stayed in my bag unless it was absolutely necessary to use it. That went on for about two years. Eventually I became its boss – I wore it when I wanted to, without feeling guilty when I didn't want to use it. Then I found I used it more and more frequently. I persevered because I could hear more. I suppose also because I could hide it under my hair, so no one needed to know.'

Joan

'My hearing loss is only slight, and I must admit, I don't use my hearing aid very much. I leave it in the drawer. The sound just doesn't sound natural. I suppose if I had to, I'd wear it more.'

Arnold

'My first hearing aid was a body worn one. I didn't like it so much because my coat used to rub against it. Now I have two privately-fitted BTE aids. They're not bad, but volume control is a problem. I was listening to a concert with a brass band and a choir, and I was forever having to fiddle with my aids, turning them up and down. Another thing with a hearing aid is that music always sounds a bit flat and out of tune. It doesn't sound like real music.'

Going private

Most people who have a hearing aid use and appreciate an NHS model. However, some people may have particular needs, or may want to try one of the latest digital aids which are only available privately. Privately-dispensed hearing aids are expensive – anything from £500 to £2,500 depending on how sophisticated the model is – so a mistake could be very costly. There are also new products, advertised in the most glowing terms, appearing on the market almost daily, and it is difficult to know where to get impartial advice. If the person you care for is considering buying a hearing aid privately, here are a few guidelines:

Choose a good dispenser. A good dispenser must be very technically skilled, because a well-fitting and finely-adjusted hearing aid will give a much better quality of sound than one which is hastily fitted. Even an expensive model can give disappointing results if it is not well fitted or adjusted to the needs of the user.

A good dispenser must also be someone who will put the interests of the patient first. Even an expensive model can give disappointing results if it is not right for the person. Most dispensers are scrupulous and honest professionals, but there is also the usual proportion of make-a-fast-buck salespeople. Word-of-mouth recommendation is always a good guide – though beware written testimonials unless you know the people who have written them. A recommendation from a GP is also useful.

If you can, accompany the person you care for when they see the private dispenser, so that you can make sure they are not put under any pressure, and that they fully understand all the details of cost and after-sales service. If the salesperson visits at home, try to be there, and remember that you have seven days in which to reconsider and change your mind.

Check the qualifications of the dispenser and make sure he or she is registered with the Hearing Aid Council (address on page 140). This is particularly important if buying through a newspaper advertisement or visiting exhibition.

Ask others. It is a good idea to ask others who have bought privately – ask members of a local deaf club, hard of hearing club or lipreading class for their opinions and advice. They will know who the reputable local dispensers are. They may also have experienced some of the advantages and disadvantages of different types of hearing aid.

If the person has already had an NHS hearing aid fitted, it is a good idea to discuss with the staff at the audiology clinic why he or she is not satisfied with their NHS aid. It may be that some quite simple adjustments could make it much better. If the staff do think that a privately-dispensed aid might be suitable, they will be able to give impartial advice.

Have a trial period. It's very important to try out a hearing aid at home and in the conditions it's going to be used in. A hearing aid which seems excellent in the quiet of the dispenser's office may be hopeless in the hustle and bustle of everyday life. Equally, someone who has not adjusted to wearing an NHS hearing aid may find it just as difficult to adjust to wearing a private aid.

Most dispensers give at least 30 days free home trial. Make sure there is a no-quibble guaranteed refund if the hearing aid is returned.

Make sure there is after-sales service. A hearing aid is bound to need tuning and adjustment from time to time, so make sure you know how this is to be carried out and how much it will cost. Make sure you know where tubing and batteries can be obtained and how much they will cost. Someone who has local premises, and has been long established in an area is likely to be easier to get hold of, and to be available for over-the-phone advice.

Tot up the cost. When working out the cost of a private hearing aid, don't forget to include insurance, maintenance and repairs, new earmoulds, tubing and batteries. Remember also that the aid will probably need to be replaced after about five years. Check whether the hearing aid is covered by the household contents insurance policy. If not, it is advisable to arrange separate insurance cover.

Read the small print. Check what guarantee is given, whether the aid can be returned if it is not satisfactory, and what happens if it goes wrong or does not function as promised.

Many people who have bought a hearing aid privately are delighted with their purchase and say it has transformed their lives, but others feel that they have wasted their money.

Madge

'When I realised I needed a hearing aid, the NHS waiting list was so long I decided to buy one privately. The one I have is digital, and it is set by computer for my particular hearing need, and can be reset as my hearing deteriorates. I am very pleased with it. The worst thing about it is the cost!'

Cleaning and maintenance

Cleaning

A behind-the-ear hearing aid should be cleaned at least once a week, by wiping it with a dry cloth or tissue. It should not be allowed to get wet, and should be kept away from direct heat.

The **earmould** should be washed every night if possible, or at least once a week. Detach the earmould gently from the hearing aid by pulling the plastic tube away from the elbow of the hearing aid (not out of the earmould). The mould should be washed in warm soapy water (not detergent), rinsed thoroughly, and left to dry in a warm (not hot) place. The tube should be washed and rinsed too, and any bits of wax removed gently with a nailbrush, then blown gently to clear any water inside.

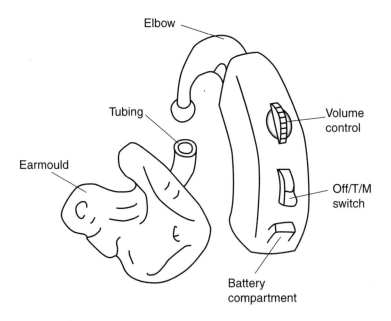

A behind-the-ear hearing aid should be wiped clean every day and the earmould washed at least once a week.
(Illustration reproduced with the permission of RNID.)

After washing, leave the earmould and tubing to dry overnight. When the earmould and tube are completely dry, they can be put back together with the hearing aid. It is important to make sure that they are put together the right way round, so that the curve on the earmould matches the curve on the hearing aid.

Note **An in-the-ear aid should NOT be washed – it should be wiped clean with a dry cloth.**

If in doubt about the care of a hearing aid, contact the audiology department or hearing aid dispenser it came from, for advice.

Changing the batteries

Free replacement batteries for NHS hearing aids can be obtained from the hearing aid centre or audiology department that fitted the hearing aid. Some GPs' surgeries, deaf clubs and lipreading classes run a battery exchange service, or there may be a postal service at the local hospital.

How long a battery lasts depends on how much it has been used and the strength of your hearing aid. It is time to change the battery when the sound starts to get faint or crackly, or the volume needs to be turned up louder than usual.

To change the battery, open the battery compartment, take out the old battery, remove the sticker from the new battery and slip it in, without forcing it. Make sure it is the right way round, with the '+' on the battery matching the '+' on the hearing aid. Do not remove the sticker from the battery before it is needed.

If the person you care for has difficulty changing the battery, perhaps because they have arthritis in their hands or sight loss, you may have to help. If it is an NHS aid, staff at the audiology department will help.

Replacing the tubing

The fine clear plastic tubing which carries the sound from the hearing aid behind the ear into the earmould will need to be replaced when it begins to harden. This can be done at the hearing aid centre that supplied it, or you can do it yourself as follows:

1   Pull the worn tubing out of the earmould and off the hearing aid elbow, and set them aside.
2   Take a new length of tubing, cut one end to a long narrow point and thread this end through the hole in the earmould.
3   Pull this end through the earmould, and measure it against the old tube to make sure it is the right length, then snip off the tapered part with a pair of scissors.
4   Use the old piece of tubing to measure the length you need for the new piece, then cut off the amount you need.
5   Reconnect to the hearing aid elbow.

If there are problems

Hearing aids are sensitive instruments, and they may need attention from time to time. Below are some common problems and their solutions. If these fail, take the hearing aid back to the clinic or the dispenser.

No sound could be due to:

- Aid not switched on, or volume too low.
- Flat battery.
- Battery put in wrong way, or sticker left on.
- Tubing has moisture in it. This could be due to condensation. Remove tubing gently and blow it out with a small puffer (see above for instructions on removing/replacing tubing).
- Earmould is dirty or blocked with wax (see page 54 for cleaning instructions).

Buzzing sound could be due to:

- Switch accidentally left in T position.
- Battery not inserted properly.
- Interference from other electrical equipment, for example fridge, television, fluorescent light.

Whistling sound could be due to:

- Earmould not put in properly.
- Tubing has a hole or is not properly attached to the elbow.
- Elbow is cracked.
- Ear wax (ask the GP to check).
- Badly fitting earmould. Try using a little *Vaseline* to seal the earmould in the ear; if this does not work, return to clinic or dispenser.

Sound is very faint. This could be due to:

- Volume control turned down.
- Moisture in the tubing (see **'No sound'** above).
- Earmould is dirty or blocked with wax (see page 54 for cleaning instructions).
- Battery is going flat.

Sound crackles or goes on and off. This could be due to:

- Faulty battery contacts. Check that the battery is in properly and the sticker has been removed.
- Faulty contacts in switch or volume control. Return to hearing aid centre or dispenser for repair.

Sound is too loud. This could be due to:

- Volume control turned up too high. Try turning it down a little. If it is still too high and the sound is uncomfortable, take it back to the hearing aid centre or dispenser to be adjusted.

For more *i*nformation

ⓘ *The NHS Hearing Aid Service*; *Buying a hearing aid*; and *Digital Hearing Aids*. Factsheets available free from RNID (address on page 142).

ⓘ *All about hearing aids* and *A user's guide to hearing aids*: booklets available from RNID.

ⓘ *How to use your hearing aid*. Booklet produced by British Telecom and available from the Department of Health at the address on page 139.

ⓘ Contact the Hearing Aid Council at the address on page 140.

5 Managing at home

Whether you live with the person you care for or are caring at a distance, you will want to reassure yourself that they are safe, secure and able to manage at home. We depend on our hearing to tell us someone is at the door, and to alert us to danger. We may use an alarm clock to wake us in the morning, and we probably like to relax in front of the TV in the evening. All of these simple things may cause problems for someone with hearing loss. However, there is plenty of technical equipment specially designed for deaf people. There is also one aid that is not very hi-tech, but can replace many of the others – a specially-trained dog.

Albert

'One of my small pleasures in life is to see people's reaction to my flashing doorbell and very loud alarm. I can see them from the kitchen window. Some have actually looked so terrified they have gone away without waiting for me to come to the door.'

Feeling at home

There is much that a person with hearing loss can do to make their home comfortable, pleasant and safe. Start by taking a look at the furnishings – too many hard bare surfaces can increase echoes and background noise. Soft furnishings, fitted carpets and thick lined curtains can make a room quieter and can eliminate echoes, making it much easier for someone with hearing loss to concentrate on the sounds they want to hear.

Getting the lighting right is important too. Harsh glaring lights, or lights that cast a strong shadow can make it harder to focus on the faces of people in the room. Half-open Venetian blinds can cast a confusing pattern of light and shade. Wallpaper with a strong bright pattern, and bright or cluttered furnishings can all add to visual distractions in the room. Soft but bright all-round lighting and soothing neutral tones can create a better environment for concentrating on people's lip patterns and facial expressions.

Technical aids can help too. A listening device incorporating a microphone and headphone can pick up sound in the room and amplify it directly into a headphone worn by the listener – ideal for people who find it difficult to follow a conversation, but who do not use a hearing aid. Many people with hearing loss now choose to fit an induction loop in one room in their house, usually the sitting room. This can be used with the T-switch on their hearing aid to amplify conversation or the television within the area covered by the loop. There is more about induction loops and other aids below.

Most aids and devices designed specially for deaf and hard of hearing people are free of VAT (Value Added Tax). An exception are video recorders that record subtitles, which carry VAT because they can also be used by hearing people.

Who's at the door?

We all know what it's like to miss a visitor because we didn't hear the doorbell. Unfortunately, if someone has hearing loss, this can happen more frequently. If the person you care for only has mild hearing loss, then you may be able to solve the problem by installing a louder doorbell. However, if this doesn't solve the problem, then there are plenty of devices with flashing lights that can tell them someone is at the door.

Some flashing light alarms show a flashing light in one room only; others are wired into the lighting circuit, and flash the lights on and off in every room when someone rings the doorbell. These are quite expensive to buy and install – in the region of £100 to £200 or more – but help may be available from social services if the deaf person meets their criteria. (See pages 123–124 for more about help from social services.)

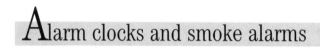

Alarm clocks and smoke alarms

If someone cannot hear an alarm clock and is regularly over-sleeping, or perhaps not getting up to let the home help in, then they may need a **vibrating alarm** to waken them. This will slip under their pillow or under the mattress. Some alarm clocks for deaf and hard of hearing people are attached to a special bedside light which flashes on and off when the telephone rings. Again, the social services department will be able to advise you, and may be able to supply the equipment.

Chris

'I have an old cheap alarm clock with a very loud bell. It's the only one I've ever found that is actually loud enough to wake me up, and I take it with me everywhere. If it ever broke down I would have to think of getting a vibrating alarm.'

It's particularly important for someone with hearing loss to have a **smoke alarm**, as they might not hear some of the sounds that would warn them of a fire, such as crackling noises and people shouting. A smoke alarm for deaf people will include a vibrating pad or a powerful strobe light or both, which will be connected by cable to the smoke detector. This means that a smoke alarm for someone with hearing loss will be much more expensive than an ordinary smoke alarm – from about £50 for a battery operated system to £150 for one that is wired into the mains electricity circuit but has a back-up battery in case the mains power supply is cut off in the fire. A whole-house system like the *Mountcastle* can also include a smoke alarm which flashes on and off with a different flash, though of course it will not necessarily alert someone who is asleep.

Arnold

'I have a smoke alarm with a flashing light and a vibrating pad under the pillow. Fortunately I've never had to use it yet, but it gives me peace of mind when I take my hearing aid out at night. When I first asked the fire officer for advice he wasn't very helpful at all. He couldn't understand why I didn't just want an alarm with a loud buzzer like everybody else.'

A home induction loop

An induction loop is a length of wire that runs around the edge of a room, starting and terminating at a control box. Also linked to this control box are one or more microphones. The microphones pick up sound and convey it to the box. The loop creates a magnetic field within which someone with a hearing aid can pick up sounds directly from the microphones by using the T-switch on their hearing aid. Background noise is eliminated, while the sounds closest to the microphone are much clearer.

Many public buildings, and counters in some shops, post offices and banks are fitted with an induction loop, but many people also have one in their own home. Some people choose to have the microphone for their induction loop placed close to the speaker of the television or radio. Others like to put the microphone close to where another person or people are sitting, so they can chat with them more easily.

If the microphone is in the middle of the room, there may be a problem if more than one person is talking, as it is impossible to tell who is speaking.

Victor

'I have an induction loop with a microphone hanging from the light. It means that anyone who comes in, I can hear them talk. I keep the television volume on ordinary, and put it on the loop. Then I put my hearing aid on the T-switch. It was money well spent.'

One major drawback with induction loops is that someone with the T-switch on can only hear sounds picked up by the microphone. They will not be able to hear the doorbell ringing or someone calling to them from another room.

You can buy an induction loop pack and install it yourself, for less than £100. It would cost more to have someone put it in for you. You can find out about firms that do installation within your area from the social services department of the council or from RNID (address on page 142).

People who do not use a hearing aid can still benefit from loop technology by buying a small listening device called a **loop listener**, which amplifies sound within the area of the loop.

Details of these and other devices are given in the RNID Sound Advantage *Solutions* catalogue (see page 67).

Enjoying television and radio

People often first realise they are going deaf when their family complain they have the television turned up too loud. If you are living with someone who has a hearing loss, you may already have experienced this. However, there are aids and devices which can enable you both to enjoy watching TV together.

Arnold

'I find people on TV are the hardest to follow. Especially comedians. They go so fast. And they move their heads from side to side when they talk, so you can't lipread. I got so fed up with missing the joke when everybody else was laughing. Now I have my TV on the loop and I can hear much better.'

Harry

'The thing that annoys me most is when people on the radio insist on talking above the music. Even with my hearing aid, I just can't make out what they're saying.'

One way of hearing the TV or radio better without turning the volume up is to use an **induction loop**, as described above. You can put the microphone for the loop close to the speaker, or even tape or clip it on. If the TV or radio has the right kind of adaptor, you can plug it directly into the loop control box, without having to use a microphone. Another way is to use a personal loop system. This is a neckloop or an earloop that is plugged into the TV or radio rather than needing a loop of wire around the room.

Another helpful device is an **infrared system**. This consists of a little transmitter which sits on top of the television or radio, and picks up the sound, either through a plug and socket connection, or through a microphone. It converts the sound into infrared light, which it beams out to anyone wearing a special receiver. The receiver then converts the light back into sound. There are two kinds of receiver, one for people who wear hearing aids, and the other for people who do not.

Like the induction loop, this system is very convenient because it means the person using it can walk around the room without trailing wires. An infrared listening system gives good sound quality, but can cost in the region of £200. One drawback is that strong sunlight can interfere with infrared systems, so you need to think carefully about where it will be sited.

Sound amplifiers work by connecting the television or radio directly by wire to the listener. An output socket or a microphone placed near to the speaker is linked to a control unit; this is linked to a headset, an earphone, or a stetoclip (see page 136) worn by the listener. Someone with a hearing aid can listen via their T-switch setting by wearing a neckloop or an earloop.

An advantage of sound amplifiers is that they are inexpensive and easy to install, as they need no special wiring. However, if the connector to the sound amplifier is plugged directly into an output socket on the TV or radio, this may cut off the sound coming out through the speakers, so no one else in the room will be able to hear it. If you live with someone who is thinking of investing in a sound amplifier, it is important to check this before you buy.

Headphones are like sound amplifiers, except that instead of linking through a control box, they are linked directly to the TV or radio. The sound quality may not be as good as an induction loop, amplifier or infrared system, and plugging the headphones in may cut off the sound through the speakers, so other people in the room will not be able to hear. However, headphones are inexpensive, easy to plug in to the TV or radio, and someone wearing them can turn the volume up as high as they want.

Listening devices can be used with a direct connection lead which plugs into a socket on the television set. This will cut down background noise such as other people talking in the room, so that all that is heard is the television. If the television doesn't have the right socket then a microphone can be fixed to the television speaker instead.

Some televisions and video recorders have a **SCART socket**. If the headset or sound amplifier has a SCART plug, it can go into this socket without cutting off the sound through the speakers, so that other people can listen too.

Teletext subtitles are especially useful for people who are severely or profoundly deaf. Many programmes now have teletext subtitles.

If your television does not have teletext, you can buy a teletext adaptor, or if the teletext is not clear you can get an aerial booster. Teletext also offers some useful 'magazine' pages especially for people who are deaf or hard of hearing, for example *Deafview* on Channel 4 and *Read Hear* on BBC2.

If the person you care for wants to use a **video recorder (VCR)**, it is important to check that it is one that records teletext subtitles. Most VCRs don't record teletext subtitles, and those that do are usually more expensive. You can buy a separate teletext decoder to attach to the VCR. If you are buying a new VCR, make sure that you actually see it working recording subtitles, and check that it can make timed recordings with subtitles. Many salespeople are not familiar with teletext subtitling, and may assume that most modern equipment has this facility without having tried it out. RNID has a factsheet, *Subtitles on TV and video*, which gives more information about VCRs that record teletext subtitles.

Pre-recorded video tapes with subtitles work differently to teletext subtitles. They are called closed-caption subtitles, and you need a separate piece of equipment, called a closed-caption decoder, to read them. Some VCRs have a built-in closed-caption decoder.

Note **Sometimes our lives get so taken over by television that it's easy to forget that we can turn it off. Remember talking to someone with hearing loss is much easier if the TV or radio is turned off.**

Hearing dogs

Everybody knows about guide dogs for the blind, but few people have seen a 'hearing dog' at work. A hearing dog can act as a doorbell, fire and smoke alarm, burglar alarm, baby alarm, and telephone bell extension. It can help you cross the road safely and help you make new friends – in fact just about the only thing it can't do is listen to the TV for you! The dog is trained to alert its owner to a significant sound by touching them with its paw, and then leading them to the source of the sound.

Like a guide dog, a hearing dog wears a distinctive yellow jacket with a logo saying 'Hearing Dog for the Deaf'. When the owner and dog go out together in public they are very visible.

Anne has a hearing dog called Rupert

'I sometimes call him my white stick. When I go out with him, it's like carrying a huge illuminated sign with me saying 'I am deaf'. I depend on lipreading to communicate, and at least when people see Rupert they know I may have trouble understanding them. It means I can be independent and it takes a lot of stress out of everyday living. I've got various gadgets to help me in the house, but once I'm out of the house, I'm lost.

'There's a social side to it, too. When people see Rupert, they stop and talk to me. I've met lots of people when I've been out with him. It's a great confidence booster.'

The dogs make good companions, and develop a very close relationship with their owner, so they continue to learn even after their period of formal training is finished. Whereas guide dogs tend to be chosen for their placid natures, hearing dogs tend to be lively, inquisitive dogs. Small or medium-sized crossbreeds are often chosen.

Before it is trained, a hearing dog spends several months with a volunteer who house-trains it and gets it used to living with people; it is then ready to learn basic commands, before being matched up with its future owner and trained to meet the owner's individual requirements. All this takes between one and two years, so unfortunately there are never enough hearing dogs to meet the needs of all the people who would like one. To qualify for a hearing dog, someone would normally have to be severely or profoundly deaf, and live on their own or with another deaf or disabled person. They would have to be a real dog lover – the special bond between the owner and the dog is what makes for a successful partnership.

Someone who is out at work all day would have to make special arrangements to take the dog to work with them. If the person you care for has another dog or dogs they can still apply, though as a general rule the hearing dog should be the only dog in the house. People who meet all these criteria may be able to get help from social services towards the cost of a hearing dog.

For more information about hearing dogs, contact Hearing Dogs for Deaf People (address on page 141).

For more *i*nformation

i Your local social services department will have information about all the different aids and adaptations mentioned here, and may be able to help towards the cost of installing them if you or the person you care for has a recognised need.

i RNID Sound Advantage is a non-profit-making marketing wing of RNID. It supplies a large range of devices and equipment for people with hearing loss, and will send a catalogue on request. All the products in the free *Solutions* catalogue have been tested, and are competitively priced. It can also give advice about products and installation (address on page 142).

i Many companies that make hearing equipment and home aids advertise regularly in the RNID members' magazine, *One in Seven*, which also contains regular features on equipment and hearing aids.

i RNID factsheets: *Doorbells for deaf people; Subtitles on TV and video; Baby alarms for deaf people; Devices to alert you to different sounds around your home; Loop systems – a guide for hearing aid users* and *Smoke alarm systems for deaf people* which review some of the equipment currently on the market. Also, RNID has booklets titled *Help with TV and audio* and *Equipment for deaf people*.

i If you use the Internet, the RNID website (www.rnid.org.uk) contains a free on-line database of equipment, to help you compare models and prices, as well as showing the factsheets and leaflets listed above.

i Contact Hearing Dogs for Deaf People at the address on page 141.

6 Using the telephone

Many carers like to keep in touch with the person they care for by telephone, but when the person has a hearing loss this can be difficult. Lipreading, and clues provided by gesture and facial expression are not possible over the telephone, so the dependence on sound is even greater. Even someone with quite a mild hearing loss may simply not hear the phone ringing, while someone with a profound hearing loss will need special equipment to allow them to communicate by phone.

Fortunately, this is one area where there is usually help available. There is a range of products on the market, and some of them may be supplied free of charge by the social services department. However, this will depend on the policy of your local authority, and varies from area to area.

Freda

'I manage quite well on the telephone, depending on who is on the other end. I have a phone which amplifies the sound, and I can also increase the volume by sliding up the bar at the bottom. We learnt about telephone technique in lipreading classes, and that was very helpful.'

Albert

'The thing I hate most is those telephone stacking systems where you have to press the button – 1,2,3 – for the service you need. At least if it's a person, you can ask them to speak slowly!'

Ringers and flashers

Someone who cannot hear the phone ring may benefit from having:

- a telephone with a different ringing tone – possibly lower. Many older people lose their hearing at the higher frequencies first, so may still be able to hear lower sounds;
- an extension telephone ringer with an extra loud ringing tone. This costs about £20, and plugs into your existing phone socket with an adaptor for the telephone;
- a telephone with a light that flashes when the telephone rings. This is useful when the telephone is on a desk where someone is working, but the flashing light will not be strong enough to alert someone who is not sitting close to the phone or keeping an eye on it;
- a flashing light telephone alerter. This could be an ordinary table light wired into the telephone through a special adaptor (this needs to be done by a qualified electrician), or it could be a special flasher unit that connects to the telephone. In each case, the light flashes on and off for an incoming call;
- a sound monitor, which picks up the sound in one room, and transmits it to a receiver in another room. This may be a receiver plugged into a mains electrical socket which uses the existing domestic wiring to transmit the sound. Or it may be a radio receiver a bit like a miniature mobile phone that the person carries around with them.

Chris

'I could never hear the telephone because the ringer sounded exactly like my tinnitus. Then I got a new telephone with a different ringing tone, and I can hear it if I'm not too far away.'

Victor

'I have a special bell for the telephone, because I couldn't hear the normal bell. It was supplied free from social services.'

Telephones and pagers

Telephones that amplify the volume

A wide range of telephones which amplify the volume of incoming speech is available from BT and from other manufacturers. The *Clarity* telephone has a sound control which can amplify sound selectively at the higher frequencies, where most hearing loss occurs. The *Converse* range of telephones can amplify both outgoing and incoming speech – useful if you frequently telephone the person you care for.

For someone who may need to use a phone away from their own home, there is even a small portable amplifier which slides onto the earpiece of an ordinary telephone. Many of these phones also have extra large keypads, making them useful for someone with sight loss, too.

More information about models and current prices is available from BT, RNID, and from the RNID Sound Advantage *Solutions* catalogue (see page 67).

Hearing aid compatible telephones

When a telephone is described as 'hearing aid compatible', it usually means it has a built-in inductive coupler (also called a loop or telecoil) in the earpiece, that works in conjunction with the T-switch on the hearing aid. When the aid is switched to the T position, and the telephone earpiece is close to that ear, the hearing aid picks up only sound from the telephone – all other sound is cut out. The sound is much clearer, and the volume can be adjusted to a comfortable level. (There is more about how an induction loop works on page 61.)

Most telephones that have a volume control also have an inductive coupler, but it is just as well to check before you buy.

Albert

'I have an induction coil and volume control on my telephone, but I tend to just use the volume control, as it is easier than switching my hearing aid to the "T".'

Listening with two ears

Some people with a hearing loss can hear much better if they are receiving the sound through both ears. This applies particularly when the T-switch is used.

Telephones with two handsets are available, but it may be cheaper just to get a telephone double adaptor plug and have two telephones connected next to each other, so the person can hold one to each ear to listen – though they will only be able to talk into one!

Telephones with built-in answering machines

Some people with hearing loss get flustered on the telephone because of the worry that they will miss something – especially if they are getting important information such as train times or meeting arrangements. Some built-in answering machines let you record the whole conversation, so it can be played back again and again.

Pagers

A pager is a useful way of getting a message to someone with a hearing loss. Many pagers have a vibrating alerter as well as a bleeper. They can store messages, and because these are viewed as text, there is no problem about hearing the message. However, they don't give the carer the instant reassurance that the other person is all right, as it is up to them to get back to you.

Textphones and Typetalk

Someone who is severely or profoundly deaf will not be able to use an ordinary telephone, even with sound amplification. In this case, a **textphone** may be the answer.

A textphone combines a keyboard like the one on a computer with a telephone receiver and a small display screen. To talk to someone by textphone, you pick up the receiver, dial, and then instead of talking, key in your message. The person at the other end picks up the receiver of their textphone and reads your words on the display screen. They may reply to you by keying in a message, or they may simply talk back. If the textphone has an ordinary handset as well as a keyboard, it can double up as a conventional telephone.

The most commonly available type of textphone in the UK is the *Minicom*, and this name is sometimes given to all textphones.

Some payphones at airports, railway stations and motorway service areas also have a textphone facility. You can find out where these are located by contacting BT on 0800 800 150 (voice) or 0800 243 123 (text).

However, to use a textphone successfully, one must have quick fingers and be familiar with a keyboard. Many older people do not get used to using a textphone, and feel much more comfortable with other communication aids, or they may use the textphone just for receiving messages. This may be because they have restricted movement in their hands due to a stroke or arthritis, or it may be because they never learnt keyboard skills, so the process of communication is painfully slow. If you are thinking of buying a textphone, the person you care for should try it out first.

John

'I tried using a Minicom once, but it didn't suit me at all. I spent ages just looking for each letter. My wife used to be a typist, so it was easy for her, and our children and grandchildren – well, you can't keep them off the computer. But it just wasn't right for me.'

Typetalk is a telephone relay service which allows deaf people who use textphones to communicate with hearing people who use telephones anywhere in the world. It currently works through an operator. The service is operated by RNID and funded by BT.

If you want to contact the person you care for by Typetalk, you call the special Typetalk number, talk to the operator, and the operator types in what you say; this is then relayed to the person's textphone, and comes up on their textphone viewing screen. They can then either type in their response to you, or speak to you directly. A new system called TextDirect will allow users to preset their account details, and to connect to Typetalk by dialling a special number. People who find typing difficult can speak to the Typetalk operator, instead of typing what they want to say.

There is no charge for the operator service, the call is charged as a direct call, and in addition the person using the textphone can claim a 60 per cent rebate, as for textphone calls (see 'Help with phone bills' below).

Deaf people who use Typetalk can also get through to the emergency services by dialling 0800 112 999.

Help with phone bills

People who use textphones or Typetalk (see above) end up with higher telephone bills, as it takes longer to key in what you want to say than it does to talk. In recognition of this, a scheme run jointly by BT and RNID can give textphone users some help with their bills. The scheme is called TURS – Text Users Rebate Scheme. It allows someone who is deaf or speech-impaired to claim a 60 per cent rebate on the cost of their phone calls, plus VAT, up to a maximum of £160 per year. To qualify, the person using the phone must:

■ be at least six years old;
■ use a textphone in their own home or a residential home;
■ be unable to use an ordinary voice phone, even with a hearing aid, an amplifier or an induction loop and T-switch.

Two hearing or speech-impaired people using the same phone still get a 60 per cent rebate, but can claim up to £320 for the year.

To claim, the person must first register on a special form, which can be obtained from BT or RNID. BT will call them at home to make sure they are textphone or Typetalk users; then they will get a letter of acceptance onto the scheme. When they have received their bill, they must pay it and then send the original bill to BT. This must be done within 16 weeks of the date on the bill.

Light user scheme

People who don't use the phone very much, or people who use their phone mainly for incoming calls, may be able to take advantage of BT's Light User Scheme. This is designed for people who spend less than a specified amount on phone calls each quarter, and it gives a rebate on the line rental if the cost of calls is below this amount. Many older people take advantage of this, but they need to register by calling BT. Dial the operator and ask for Customer Services.

BT and other telecom companies have various other payment schemes and services available to all their customers. You can get information about these from your telecom company's Customer Services.

The Internet

The Internet provides a wonderful means of communication for people with hearing loss. Sending and receiving messages is almost immediate, and a whole world of information is available at your fingertips. A number of websites of special interest to people with hearing loss are listed under 'Useful Addresses' at the end of this book.

There are many Internet Service Providers (ISPs) who provide both a line to the World Wide Web and support and information for users. Unfortunately, if things go wrong they tend to provide help by telephone. Technology being developed now means that people can access the Internet from home through their television, as well as through a computer.

Many household names provide Internet services, and these are advertised widely in newspapers and magazines.

For more *i*nformation

- *i* The social services department of your local authority will be able to tell you what telephones are available, and what help may be available free of charge in your area.

- *i* *The BT guide for disabled people: the latest products and services* booklet available free of charge. For this and other helpful information, telephone 0800 800 150 (voice) or 0800 243 123 (textphone).

- *i* To find out more about Typetalk, telephone 0800 7311 888.

- *i* RNID produces the booklets, *Telephones* and *Typetalk*, and also a series of leaflets describing the Typetalk service and how to use it.

- *i* The *Solutions* catalogue produced by RNID Sound Advantage (address on page 142) contains a number of telephones and textphones.

7 Getting out and about

People with hearing loss often say that one of the hardest things they have to cope with is their loss of confidence in social situations. This is not surprising when you discover how much rudeness and intolerance they have to face. It's all too easy to let this become a barrier to getting out and about. However, most people are not deliberately rude – they just don't know how to be helpful.

There is much you can do as a carer to make communication easier when you go out with someone who has hearing loss. There is also much they can do to help themselves when they go out alone. People with hearing loss describe some of the problems and anxieties they face in everyday situations, which are difficult for a person with normal hearing to imagine.

Harry

'Years ago, people used to think being deaf was the same as being stupid. Deaf and dumb, they would say. There's still a bit of it about. I was out shopping one day, and a chap stopped and asked me something. He was mumbling and talking quite fast. Well, I just didn't get it, so I asked him to repeat it. He said it again, even faster, so I asked him to repeat it again. The third time I asked him, he just swore at me and walked off. That kind of thing is very upsetting.'

Overcoming prejudice

It's important not to let an experience like Harry's stop you and the person you care for from enjoying life to the full. Remember, most people are helpful and sympathetic once they realise someone has a hearing loss. They are simply not aware that many people they meet every day are deaf or hard of hearing, and they do not know how best to communicate.

Sometimes, however, thoughtless remarks can really hurt.

Pauline

'When Mum went deaf, our youngest sister was still at school. She found it very hard to cope with Mum's deafness – she felt as though Mum was rejecting her when she didn't respond. We had to keep explaining that Mum loved her, but she just couldn't hear what she was saying. She had quite a traumatic time. One day, the teacher at school said something to her, and she took no notice. So the teacher said, "What's the matter? Are you deaf or are you stupid?" Well, she just went absolutely bananas.'

As a carer of someone with hearing loss, you have an important role in helping re-educate society about the way people with hearing loss are seen. You may be able to speak up where the person with hearing loss feels too embarrassed. Speaking up doesn't mean you have to be unpleasant or make a fuss. Sometimes gentle persuasion is more effective.

Joan

'I have "deaf awareness" now, but I didn't before. When we go out together, I always speak up for him. If we go to the cinema or the theatre, and there isn't a loop system I always mention to them how much more my husband would have enjoyed it.'

Sometimes the hardest thing to do is also the most useful, as Madge (below) found: admitting to having a hearing loss, and asking the other person to repeat or speak more clearly.

Madge

'I don't find a problem. I am quite active at church and enjoy theatre-going, and in both places they have a loop system. If I don't hear what people say I ask them to repeat and explain that I'm hard of hearing. I remember once being out in a group, and mishearing what someone said, and answering wrongly. Someone in the group laughed at me and I was very hurt, but the lady saw it and apologised. I have had very few bad experiences – frustrating ones sometimes.'

Be prepared

Each individual with hearing loss has different communication needs. How does the person you care for prefer to communicate – by sign language, lipreading, using a hearing aid, or a combination of these? By thinking ahead, and helping the person you care for to plan some of the communication in advance, you can help take much of the stress out of a situation.

People with hearing loss often don't have the confidence to say what they want to say – they feel they must wait until they're spoken to. Then they have the stress and anxiety of struggling to make out what is said and how to respond. No wonder they get disheartened. A different approach is to go into a situation having already decided what they want to say. Taking control of a situation in this way can be a real confidence booster. The key is to be well prepared.

Sounding out the situation

If someone knows what they want to say, they don't need to wait for the other person to speak. Most situations are fairly predictable –

it's not difficult to work out what questions will be asked and what words will be used. In many situations, the person with hearing loss can prepare what it is he or she wants to say, and take control of the situation. Of course, there will always be an element of unpredictability, but by planning ahead that can be kept to a minimum.

The situation

- Will it be indoors or outdoors?
- Will it involve talking to people in a group, or face-to-face conversation with one person?
- Will the room have an induction loop?
- What sort of background noise will there be?
- Will there be a quiet room to slip away to?
- What will the lighting be like?

The conversation

- What will the other person want to say to the person with hearing loss?
- Will they need to catch the person's attention?
- What questions will be asked?
- What words will be used?
- Are any of the words confusing to lipread?
- What are the key points the person with hearing loss wants to get across?
- What is the key information they need to come away with?

You can help the person you care for to be prepared by going through some of these points with them before they go out.

Signs to look out for

Induction loop

Many public places are now fitted with an induction loop. You will usually find at least one counter at the bank, building society, post office, railway station ticket office and many shops, has a small induction loop. This is just a coil of wire that starts and ends at a control box amplifier. When the control box is switched on, a magnetic field is set up, and every sound inside this field is picked up by a special microphone

Most hearing aids have a special switch setting called the T position, to pick up sounds directly from the microphone, and completely cut out background noise. Look out for the induction loop sign below to find out if there is a loop available. If there is a loop available, check that it is working and switched on. If the person you care for finds that the loop does not help, tell the staff working at the venue. See page 48 to find out more about the T-switch.

Look out for this sign. It means an induction loop is installed.
(Illustration reproduced from RNID *All about hearing aids*.)

Sympathetic Hearing Scheme

As you can see from reading Chapter 3, communicating with someone with hearing loss needs care and patience. Most people have little awareness of the problems deaf and hard of hearing people face, unless they have some personal experiences to make them aware. The Sympathetic Hearing Scheme, run by the charity Hearing Concern, trains people who deal with the public in how to communicate with people who have a hearing loss. Many large organisations that deal with the public now send staff on these training courses. The sign below indicates that a member of staff in the building has been on a Sympathetic Hearing course. However, they may not realise that the person they are talking to has a hearing loss, unless that person wears a badge, shows them a card or tells them.

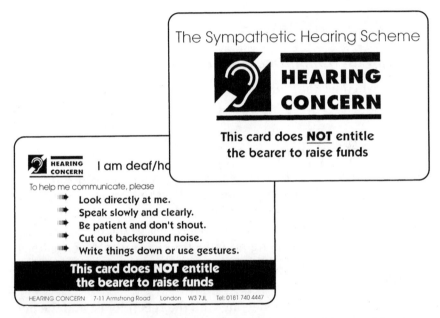

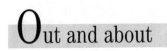

Sympathetic Hearing Scheme card – showing this card invites others to show consideration.
(Illustration reproduced by permission from Hearing Concern.)

For more information, contact the Sympathetic Hearing Scheme, Hearing Concern, at the address on page 140.

Out and about

When you go out and about with someone who has a hearing loss, you soon become aware of factors which can make communication harder or easier for them. There are environmental factors such as lighting and acoustics, and there are ways of managing the conversation itself by predicting and preparing for some of the things which are most likely to be said. The common situations discussed below show how useful it is to be prepared.

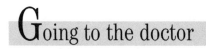

Going to the doctor

Making an appointment by telephone

Check whether the surgery has a textphone, or knows about Typetalk.

The reception area

Some doctors' surgeries are fitted with an induction loop, and some doctors will employ a sign language interpreter if they are given enough notice. Unfortunately, these are the exception rather than the rule. You might feel able to suggest to the doctor or practice manager that installing an induction loop would be relatively inexpensive, and could benefit many of their patients who use a hearing aid.

On the positive side, the meeting with the receptionist and the doctor will be individual and face to face, and it should be possible to prepare in advance some things to say.

The situation

First the reception/waiting room. This will be fairly quiet, but if the person has to wait to see the doctor, they may not hear when their name is called. The receptionist may be sitting on a lower level than the patient, and may be looking down when she talks. There may even be a glass screen. This does not make for good communication.

Margaret

'There was a new practice nurse last time I went to the surgery, so I introduced myself and told her I've got a hearing problem. She said "That makes two of us, then." Then she sat down at her computer, and only turned her head towards me from time to time. Most of the time I could only see the side of her mouth when she talked to me. She had no idea how to communicate.'

The conversation

However, the conversation at reception will be fairly straightforward. The receptionist will want to know the patient's name, the time of the appointment, and which doctor they are seeing. This is information the patient can volunteer – they don't have to wait to be asked. They will need to tell the receptionist that they cannot hear when their name is called, they will need to be alerted. Some GPs also have a visual alerting system so a deaf person can see when it is their turn.

Chris

'I hate reception desks with a high counter and things on it which obstruct my view of the person's face. I really hate it when they call names over a tannoy system. When I'm sitting in the waiting room, I have to watch when they call the names to make sure someone has got up – otherwise it could be me! I can't concentrate on reading a magazine – I have to concentrate on making sure I don't miss my turn. It's an extra stress at a time when I'm feeling stressed and under-the-weather already.'

In the doctor's surgery

The situation

Again, this will be quiet, and there will be just one person for the patient to talk to. Some doctors have a habit of looking down when they talk, and the light may be in the wrong place. Think about the best place to sit, and if necessary encourage the person to move their chair.

Rene

'When I went in to see the doctor this morning he greeted me by my name, then he moved away from his desk, sat down facing me and said, "Now, you tell me all about it." I thought, after we all complain about doctors so much, I should be grateful my doctor is so considerate.'

The conversation

The doctor will start with a greeting and invite the patient to describe the problem. This will be the cue for the patient to describe what's wrong. That's the easy part – the part you and the person you care for have prepared in advance. After this, the conversation becomes more difficult. It's important to understand the doctor's questions – guessing and giving the wrong answer could have serious consequences, so be prepared to ask the doctor to repeat things, and even to write them down. Some doctors, like Rene's, are aware of the problems deaf and hard of hearing people face. Others, even ENT (ear, nose and throat) consultants, sometimes forget, and carry on talking while writing or looking at papers.

Chris did some training for the Sympathetic Hearing Scheme

'I gave a talk to the staff at the GP's surgery about communicating with people with hearing loss. The nurses and receptionists came, but none of the doctors came.'

One way a carer can help is to make sure the surgery makes a note on the patient's notes, to indicate that he or she has a hearing loss, and their preferred way of communicating, such as by lipreading, sign language interpreter or using their hearing aid.

If a patient is to be referred to a specialist, you can ask the GP to make sure they highlight the patient's communication needs, so the specialist can be prepared.

Going into hospital

If the person you care for has to go into hospital, it's very important that the professionals caring for them know about their hearing loss. When someone goes into hospital, their initial assessment should note any communication needs they have, so that these are available to the ward charge nurse. If you think the special problems of the person you care for have not been noted, mention this to the charge nurse.

If someone is having treatment or surgery in an ENT (ear, nose and throat) department, then the ward staff will be familiar with the needs of people with hearing loss. But in general wards, the ward staff may be less aware of the needs of deaf patients. Everyone who comes into contact with the patient, from doctors and nurses, to therapists, to tea and dinner ladies, needs to know that they have a hearing loss, and that they should take the time and trouble to communicate with them.

John

'We all know how awful it is to lie in a hospital bed while the consultant discusses our case with the nurse or lectures a group of medical students. Imagine how much worse it is when you know they are talking about you, but you can't hear what they're saying.'

Judith

'My mother found the hospital experience very distressing. She couldn't tell when they were talking to her unless they touched her or called her name. They would offer her a cup of tea or something to eat, and if she didn't respond, they would assume she didn't want anything.'

Many hospitals now have specialist units or specialist staff who liaise with the ward and clinical staff, to make sure that the needs of patients with hearing loss are recognised and catered for. Special provision for people with hearing loss in hospital could include:

■ sign language interpreters or lipspeakers (these will need to be booked well in advance, so make sure the ward charge nurse is alerted);

■ access to a textphone, so that someone with hearing loss can communicate with a partner or carer who has a textphone;

■ a loop on the ward, or a portable loop that can be brought to the ward for someone who uses a hearing aid;

■ TV with teletext so they can use subtitles (see page 64);

■ training for staff on how to communicate with patients with a hearing loss.

Using a hearing aid in hospital

You should inform the charge nurse if the person you care for uses a hearing aid, and explain any particular difficulties. Ask if there is a loop system on the ward, or if a portable loop can be brought in. Make sure that the person you care for can get their hearing aid, and that there is a safe convenient place to put it when they take it out. It is easy for someone to lose their hearing aid in the hustle and bustle of a busy ward – it may have been picked up by mistake by another patient, or it may have fallen into the bed and got bundled up with the bed linen when it was being changed. If this happens, make sure the charge nurse is alerted at once, so that it can be traced – especially if it is an expensive private one. You should also make sure that the person you care for has their private hearing aid insured against loss.

Shopping

The situation

Shops can be noisy, busy places with variable lighting and lots of visual distraction. Some larger stores have induction loops fitted, and some have staff trained to listen under the Sympathetic Hearing Scheme – look out for a sign by the entrance door (see pages 80–81).

This means that someone on the staff has been on a special training course to teach them how to communicate with someone who has a hearing loss, covering many of the points made in Chapter 3.

Chris

'I don't find shopping a problem, except where sums of money are stated. I'm OK if I can see the amount on the till. Greengrocers' shops can be difficult because the till is often underneath the scales. And staff in sandwich shops have an annoying habit of talking while facing the back wall as they prepare the sandwiches.'

The conversation

Fortunately, it's easy to take control of the conversation when you're shopping, just by asking for what you want. Gestures and pointing can replace words, but it may be helpful to alert the shop assistant to the fact that someone cannot hear what they say.

Merryl

'Mum and Dad always used to take notes rather than coins with them when they went shopping. Then when the shop assistant said how much something cost, they would hand over the money and wait for the assistant to give them the change. It saved them from the embarrassment of having to admit they couldn't hear. Of course supermarkets have changed all that. Everything's displayed on shelves, so you don't have to ask, and the cost is displayed at the till so you can watch the price of goods being clocked up. They're much better for deaf people.'

'When I go shopping, I often have to say to people, "I'm sorry, I can't hear you, can you say that again". Now I have a little badge that says "Hard of Hearing. Please speak clearly."'

Some larger shops, such as supermarkets and DIY stores, have introduced induction loops at the tills and have staff trained to be deaf aware. Ask at the customer information desk about any special services.

The hairdresser

For many people, going to the hairdresser is an opportunity to relax and enjoy a chat as well as having their hair done. However, people with a hearing loss can find a visit to the hairdresser particularly stressful. Lots of bare hard surfaces, humming dryers and running water can make for a noisy and confusing environment. If they wear a hearing aid, they will have to take it out. As for lipreading – imagine trying to lipread somebody who is standing behind you, and whose face you can only see in the mirror.

Some people find that having a hairdresser visit them at home makes for a more relaxed atmosphere. However, a visit to the hairdresser can still be an enjoyable experience if the person with hearing loss takes the initiative from the start, and explains what they want, rather than waiting to be asked.

Banks and building societies

Doreen

'I got so frustrated at the building society branch. It's bad enough having to speak through a glass screen. But the assistant was seated below me, and she was looking down reading out figures from a sheet in front of her. I couldn't hear, and I couldn't see her face. I had to ask her to repeat three times.'

The situation

Understanding someone talking through a glass screen can be particularly difficult for a person with hearing loss. Larger banks and building societies usually have at least one counter position fitted with an induction loop, and it should be marked with the induction loop logo. Even if there is no sign, it's always a good idea to ask. Most banks and building societies do have a quiet interview room where someone can go if they have something to talk about which can't be discussed at the counter. Many banks and building societies have also had some of their staff members trained under the Sympathetic Hearing Scheme.

However, one bank representative was frank about the problems:

'Yes, we do have an induction loop on at least one counter. We used to have sticky labels to show which one, but those have long since disappeared. Then we had stand-up signs but they aren't always on display. And yes, we did send staff on Sympathetic Hearing Scheme training courses, but we were told that a deaf or hard of hearing person would wear a special badge or carry a card. In practice, we find deaf people don't want to draw attention to themselves, they just want to get on with their life like everybody else does. But if someone asks, we will always do our best to help.'

As a carer, you can ring up and enquire which branches of the bank or building society do have induction loops, and which have trained and sympathetic staff. If the local branch is not up to scratch, do have a word with the manager and try to persuade him or her to have one installed. Most large financial institutions are very keen to have a sympathetic and customer-friendly image. If the person you care for can use their bank or building society without needing to have someone go with them, it will be a great boost to their independence and self-confidence.

The conversation

It's a good idea to work out exactly what someone wants to achieve from a visit to the bank or building society. Usually it's a straightforward request that can be prepared in advance. If it's a question requiring a complex answer, then the person should ask to be shown into an interview room, where they will be able to talk in private. They will also be sitting facing the person dealing with their query, and will feel less embarrassed if they have to ask for something to be repeated. Having to shout out your private business at a public counter can be very humiliating.

Places of worship

Many places of worship nowadays are fitted with induction loops. If the person you care for attends one that does not, then ask if a loop could be installed. The chances are, there will be a number of people who would welcome it.

The situation

Many places of worship are large echoey buildings, with high ceilings, lots of hard bare surfaces and dim or angled light. Wonderful for music and singing, but not for hearing what someone is saying. The face of the person speaking may not be clearly visible, and even with an induction loop it may not be easy to follow what is said.

Chris

'I always hope there will be a loop – otherwise I might as well not bother to attend the service. And I try to make sure it's switched on before the service. I go out to many churches testing their loops and giving advice about how to operate them properly. I often find it's the way they are operated that causes problems, rather than the loop itself.'

'My Grandad doesn't bother with his hearing aid at the mosque because he knows what's going on, and even if he can't hear the words, he likes to feel he's taking part.'

The conversation

Much of the religious service will be familiar and predictable – that is part of the beauty of it – and someone with hearing loss can still take part. However, hearing the sermon and any special prayers and announcements is going to be difficult unless there is a loop system. The acoustics of the building may produce some strange effects in a hearing aid.

Going out for a meal

When you go out for a meal with the person you care for, choosing the right setting in which you can enjoy a pleasant conversation may take precedence over the quality of the menu – though of course you may have a favourite restaurant that offers both.

The situation

Many restaurants nowadays favour a busy and noisy atmosphere with bare floors, walls and wipe-down tables, clattering of crockery and cutlery, lots of banging and shouting from the kitchen, a loud hubbub of conversation, and maybe even background music to boot. This kind of setting is pure torture to someone who uses a hearing aid. The traditional restaurant with thick carpet, wallpaper, curtains and tablecloths and quiet waiters may be a much better choice.

Most restaurants have difficult lighting as well – candlelight is fine for romance, but not so good for lipreading! You may have to ask for the candle on the table to be taken away, and the main lighting to be turned up a bit. If there is background music, choose a table well away from the speakers, or better still, ask for it to be turned down.

Remember that it is difficult for someone with a hearing loss to hold a conversation and eat at the same time. They need to concentrate on what is being said to them, which means watching the face of the person talking. While they do this, they are likely to have to stop eating. Also, it's not easy or pleasant to try and lipread someone else who is eating. The best solution is to stop talking and eat for a few minutes, then resume the conversation for a while, then stop talking and eat again.

Chris

'I often find that by the time I get to eat my food, it's cold. If you lipread, then you have to be watching the other person while they're talking, so you can't be getting on with your own food.'

If you are going out with a group of people, maybe to celebrate, then think about the shape and dimensions of the table.

Chris

'I've learned from bitter experience that a long table with people seated down both sides is hopeless for someone with hearing loss. You are sideways on to the people closest to you, so you have to keep asking them to turn their heads when they talk, while the person facing you is too far away to hear amid the hubbub of conversation. A round table is better, where you can see everyone. Nowadays when we go out as a group, we ask for separate tables to be set in fours.'

The conversation

It may be possible to look at the menu and decide exactly what to order. However, it's where choices come in that problems can arise. What is the soup of the day? What kinds of desserts are on offer? Large or small portions? All of these are likely to cause problems unless the waiter is a skilled communicator. The vocabulary may be unfamiliar – especially if it's a restaurant that specialises in foreign cuisine. Have a pen and notepad handy and be prepared to ask the waiter to write down any words that are not clear.

Talking with friends over the dinner table may be difficult too. A quiet restaurant can be a good place for a one-to-one conversation with someone, especially if they can lipread. But trying to keep up conversation with a number of different people can be very stressful for someone with hearing loss. Someone with hearing loss may prefer not to try to talk to everyone at the same time, or to join in the general conversation, but to concentrate on enjoying one-to-one talks.

Margaret

'I have to make sure I'm not sitting on the wrong side of the person I want to talk to. I have some hearing in one ear, but the other ear is completely deaf.'

Going to the theatre or cinema

Most large cinemas and theatres have induction loops, so hearing the show is not a problem for a lot of hearing aid users. The induction loop may not cover the whole auditorium, it may only be available in certain seats, so it's important to mention it when booking the tickets, particularly for very popular shows where all the seats need to be pre-booked. Many cinemas and theatres also have an induction loop or microphone system at the box office counter.

Of course, once the hearing aid is switched to the T position, then the person will not be able to hear anything at all that is not being transmitted by the induction loop – so don't bother asking them to pass the popcorn!

93

Smaller, local and amateur theatres and cinemas will probably not have an induction loop, so it's important to check before booking. Otherwise a person with hearing loss may not be able to follow the performance at all.

Joan

'We went to a pantomime at the community hall. It was great fun, but Harry couldn't hear a thing. After the show, I went up to them and said, "It's such a shame you haven't got an induction loop. My husband wears a hearing aid, and he missed all the dialogue. It would only cost about £100 to have a loop put in." I suppose they think it's not worth it with it being such a small place, but I always make a point of mentioning it wherever I go.'

Social occasions and parties

Many deaf and hard of hearing people dread parties and social occasions. Whereas staff in shops and offices may have been trained to be polite and patient, often unfortunately one's own family and friends have not.

Chris

'Social occasions are often a nightmare. The worst thing is being introduced to new people – I can never be sure I've caught their names. I try to talk to just one or two people at a time, rather than joining in a group conversation. Many people expect you to be able to follow any speech by lipreading, whatever the environment or background noise, and they make you feel foolish when you can't.'

The situation

Social occasions are usually noisy – for hearing people that all adds to the atmosphere. But for someone with hearing loss it just adds to the stress. Those who use a hearing aid will find the background noise is amplified as well as the foreground noise. Those who depend on lipreading will find they are having to watch too many different people, who may be moving about, turning their heads, wearing distracting clothes or jewellery and standing in poor light.

Chris

'There's no easy answer. Turning off the hearing aid is not a solution – it's like putting an earplug in. It's better to turn it right down. However, you don't want to embarrass yourself by constantly fiddling with the volume on your hearing aid. If the amplification of background noise is a real problem, it's better to take the hearing aid out altogether. A normal ear, even one that's hard of hearing, will discriminate between foreground and background noise, but a hearing aid will not.

'The latest digital hearing aids claim they can tune in to the sound of the voice, but it's not necessarily the voice of the person you're speaking to, if there's other loud voices in the background. They're now working on a digital hearing aid that will distinguish between a foreground voice and voices in the background. But even if they do bring it in – it will be too expensive for most people.'

The conversation

Another problem with parties is that you never know what people are going to be talking about – of course that's partly why we go. Whether it's the latest gossip, or the latest joke, or just catching up with news, it's impossible to predict what people are going to say – and that makes joining in so much more difficult for someone with hearing loss.

95

Gillian

'One thing I really hate is when I'm talking to people, and I miss something so I ask them to repeat it, and they say, "Oh, it doesn't matter". It matters to me. I can hear them all laughing but I don't know what they're laughing at.'

Some people with hearing loss admit that they find the whole business so frustrating that they tend to withdraw into themselves and avoid social situations. If you see this happening to the person you care for, don't just cajole them or tell them to cheer up. The chances are you will make them even more unhappy and self-conscious. Try to discuss it with them, and think of ways of making a social occasion enjoyable for them, for example by making sure that there are enough people who will sit and talk to them face to face and not make them feel left out.

Arnold

'If you're in a gathering and someone in the room has a very loud voice, you don't hear the person you're talking to, you just hear that voice. The noisiest place in Sheffield is the Central Deaf Club, because everyone talks too loud!'

Travelling by bus and train

When we travel, we rely on our hearing to provide us with all sorts of vital information. Someone with hearing loss will have to learn to rely on visual clues. They will probably be able to manage quite well on familiar routes, but may run into difficulties when they set out on unfamiliar journeys.

For example, travel by bus is fine if someone knows where they are going, and knows how much the fare is. But if they have to rely on the driver to tell them, they may not hear the fare, and they may not hear when their stop is called. Buses with a conductor are better, but these are rare outside London.

Merryl

'Mum and Dad used to manage on the bus by handing over a note and relying on the driver to give them the right change. But not all bus companies will accept that. And they would always sit near the front, so they could see if he was calling them for their stop, because if they sat near the back they wouldn't be able to hear.'

Rail journeys present similar problems. Finding out about train times and booking the tickets can be done by telephone. Most railway companies now have a textphone service for information and bookings (see pages 72–73 for more about textphones). The number will be in the local telephone directory under 'Railways'. For people who book at the station, the booking office should have at least one position fitted with an induction loop, so look out for the sign.

The situation

Railway stations, with their noise and bustle and vast echoing platforms, can be very stressful for someone with hearing loss. However, there will be plenty of visual clues. Details of trains and platforms are usually on display, and arrivals and departures will also be displayed on a board or screen, both in the main hall and also on individual platforms.

Problems arise when last minute changes are announced over the public address system. Most people find tannoy announcements difficult to follow; someone with a hearing loss doesn't stand a chance. The secret is to watch – watch the reactions of other travellers, watch out for any sudden large movements of people which suggest that there has been a change of platform. Then ask a helpful person, preferably someone in a railway uniform, which platform the train is leaving from. If the answer isn't clear, get them to write it down.

You might think that once the person was on the train all their problems would be over. Far from it. Announcements made on the train over the loudspeaker system completely ignore the needs of people with a hearing loss. They may just miss out on a free cup of tea or coffee, or the name of the train steward. Worse, they may find themselves in the wrong part of the train if the train divides, or they may miss an announcement about changes of stops, times, and destinations. Someone who can hear that there has been an announcement but can't make out what was said can at least ask other passengers. Someone who doesn't realise that an announcement has been made at all can miss their destination. No wonder many people with hearing loss say they find travel very stressful.

Helen

'I'd been down to Kent to visit my daughter. On the way back, the front half of the train went to London, while the back half of the train went straight up to Luton. Luckily, one of the other passengers was able to explain to me what was happening, and I quickly had to get off and run down the platform. I nearly ended up missing my connection.'

The conversation

There is just one piece of information the hearing impaired traveller needs to repeat. That is his or her destination. Staff will be able to indicate the platform number and time, and point the way. Rather than asking a question which requires an answer, for example 'Which platform does the Luton train go from?', it is better to ask, 'Is this the train to Luton?' or 'Can you show me where the Luton train goes from?'.

Help for people with hearing loss

Most railway companies make provision for people with disabilities, including someone with hearing loss. You can ask for travel assistance at the same time as you book the ticket (see 'For more information' on page 101). You may need to fill in a form detailing the person's needs. This means they will be met at the platform, and staff will make sure they get safely on the train. The train manager, steward or conductor will walk down the train at least once, and someone with hearing loss should make themselves known, and ask to be kept informed of any announcements.

Of course what happens in an ideal world is not always the same as the experience that passengers who have a hearing loss report. If the person you care for experiences any problems, it's important to report them. Things will only get better if those who provide a service are informed when it doesn't work properly.

Look out for danger

People with a hearing loss may be at risk when they are out and about, because so many danger signals in our environment rely on sound. If someone has recently lost their hearing, then they may be particularly at risk, as they will have to look out for other warning clues.

Pauline

'Mum was completely deaf, so she relied on the Green Man signal to tell her when to cross the road. Once, when she was out, she came up to a crossing, and because the Green Man was showing, she stepped out into the road. At that moment, a fire engine came past with its blue lights flashing. Its siren must have been going full blast, too, but she couldn't hear it at all. A moment later and she would have been dead.'

Albert

'I was on a cruise holiday once, and I woke up one morning to find the ship was completely empty. Eventually I found where everyone was – they were all up on the deck with their blankets around them. The fire alarm had gone off, but of course I take my hearing aids out at night, so I didn't hear a thing.'

There is always a balance to be struck between putting someone at risk, or protecting them so much that their quality of life is impoverished. If you are worried that the person you care for is taking too many risks, it may be better to get another professional, such as a social worker or hearing therapist to talk to them. If you try to protect them yourself, it may seem to them that you are interfering.

Facing up to discrimination

Under the new Disability Discrimination Act, it is against the law to discriminate against people with a disability such as hearing loss. The law covers four main areas:

- provision of goods and services
- employment
- public transport
- housing

In each of these areas, it is unlawful for someone with a disability to be treated differently from any other member of the public. Businesses, service providers and employers have to be able to show that they are taking steps to end discrimination. If the person you care for thinks they have been denied access to a product or service because of their hearing loss, they may have grounds for complaint. Contact RNID or your local Citizens Advice Bureau for advice, or ring the Disability Rights Commission Helpline on 0845 7622 633.

For more *i*nformation

i *How to cope with hearing loss* is a very useful video showing how someone with hearing loss can cope and take control in everyday situations. It is available from Lipservice at the address on page 141, price £19.

i Contact Hearing Concern at the address on page 140.

i Rail travel: Each separate railway company makes its own arrangements for helping people with disabilities. There is no central number. For textphone numbers, Customer Services and Disabled Travel Assistance numbers, look in the local telephone directory. Alternatively, ring the main timetable enquiries number, 0845 748 4950 or textphone 0845 605 0600, and they will be able to give you the number for the rail company for the journey you want to make. People who use the internet can visit Railtrack's website; www.railtrack.co.uk, to find out about train times.

8 Tinnitus and other conditions

People with hearing loss may suffer from a number of other distressing conditions. Sometimes, as in the case of tinnitus or balance problems, these originate in the ear itself. But sometimes, as with Alzheimer's disease or depression, it is the psychological effects of hearing loss that are relevant.

If you are caring for a person with hearing loss who also has other medical conditions, you need to consider how one may affect the other. For example, visits to the doctor or hospital for some completely unrelated ailment may pose particular problems for someone with hearing loss.

Madge

'Apart from my deafness, I have osteoporosis, dizziness, hypertension and some visual impairment which is getting much worse. My hearing is only one of these irritations. As yet I don't think it has added to them or made them more difficult to cope with, but I feel that my ear problems and dizziness could be connected.

'I have always been a very active person, and find it hard to accept that I am not able to do as much.'

Tinnitus

Tinnitus is the name we give to sounds we hear in our ears or head which have no apparent source in the outside world. Many people who have a hearing loss also have tinnitus. Like hearing loss, it can be caused by exposure to loud noise, by infection, by other damage to the ear, or just by ageing. Sometimes there is no obvious cause.

What does tinnitus sound like?

Most of us have experienced tinnitus from time to time. After we've been in a very noisy environment, such as a disco, we may hear a ringing, buzzing or hissing sound in our ears for some time afterwards. Or sometimes when we are in a very quiet environment we become aware of sounds our body makes which we are not aware of most of the time. For some people with tinnitus, the noises are intrusively loud – and they do not go away.

Harry

'I'm always aware of my tinnitus – it's like a bell clanging at the back of my head.'

Chris

'I hear a permanent ringing noise, like the tone of a telephone. I had to get a new telephone with a different tone to my tinnitus.'

Arnold

'I lost my hearing in the war. All I can hear in my right ear is my tinnitus. It's a loud hissing sound, like the sound of steam escaping from a pipe at high pressure. I hear it all the time. It's always there.'

Gillian

'I have had tinnitus all my life for as long as I can remember, so it's become part of my life. If you like, it's just me! It's the first thing I hear on waking and the last thing before I sleep at night. I try to keep myself busy so I can push the noises into the back of my mind, but they don't go away. Nothing is ever silent. I went to a Roman fort on Hadrian's wall with my son last year. It was late afternoon, high on the hillside. No one else was around. My son said, "Just listen to all that quiet!" But, of course, to me there were still those wretched noises in my head.'

Help with tinnitus

Sometimes tinnitus has an obvious cause, such as an ear infection, a build up of ear wax, or a reaction to some forms of medication. In these cases, the tinnitus will be 'cured' by a course of antibiotics, or by having the ear wax removed, or when the course of medication is completed.

Often, however, there is no known cure for tinnitus. But that does not mean nothing can be done about it. As we have become more aware of the problems that tinnitus can cause, there has been more research into ways of alleviating the symptoms.

Unfortunately, some GPs do not realise just how much help there is available for people with tinnitus. This is where your powers of gentle persuasion may be needed. If the GP does not offer any help, ask him or her to refer the person you care for to the audiology clinic, where the staff will be more aware of the treatments that are available.

Gillian

'The first GP I saw for my tinnitus dismissed the problem. He said there was nothing they could do and I'd just have to get used to it.'

Counselling

People with tinnitus sometimes react with annoyance when they are offered counselling for their tinnitus. They know their problem is physical in origin, not psychological, and they think accepting counselling means admitting they have a psychological problem. But the right kind of counselling can help someone to cope better with their tinnitus, so it does not dominate their life.

If the person you care for is offered counselling, try to encourage them to go along. The sessions are usually very informal – they may not even realise they are being 'counselled' – and they will almost certainly come away feeling better about themselves, and with a few strategies for managing to live with their tinnitus.

Learning to relax

Most people with tinnitus will say that their tinnitus gets worse when they are under stress. Learning to relax can help push tinnitus to the back of the mind: it is still there, but it's not bothersome.

There may be special relaxation classes they can attend, or a tinnnitus clinic may be able to lend out relaxation tapes. Some people find alternative therapies such as yoga or acupuncture or aromatherapy very relaxing. Avoiding stress but keeping the mind occupied are the twin goals to aim for.

Doreen

'I was told my tinnitus could have been caused by arthritis in my neck following a whiplash injury. If I'm under stress my tinnitus gets much worse, particularly if anyone who also suffers mentions it. I hardly notice it if I'm concentrating on something else I enjoy, such as reading or gardening. Thankfully, it doesn't affect my sleep.'

If sleep is a problem, as it is for many people with tinnitus, offer these suggestions to the person you care for:

- Take regular exercise.
- Take time to relax and unwind in the evening; don't work or exercise too late.
- Have a hot milky drink or a cup of camomile tea before bed.
- Avoid tea or coffee, especially within two hours of bed time.
- Make sure the room is quiet, dark and well-ventilated.
- A radio playing softly through a pillow-speaker or a personal stereo can help take their mind off the tinnitus.

RNID has produced two audio tapes: *Tinnitus Stress Management* and *Tinnitus Surf Sounds*, available from the address on page 142.

Medication

Some doctors will prescribe medication for anxiety or sleep loss connected with tinnitus, but there is no medication to stop the tinnitus itself.

Masking noise

Some people find that a busy environment with some background noise makes their tinnitus much more bearable. For example, leaving a window open to traffic sounds, or having the radio on, or special tapes that play soothing natural sounds, can make tinnitus seem less intrusive. But if these are not effective, it may be helpful to use a noise generator (formerly called a tinnitus masker). This is like a hearing aid, but instead of amplifying sound it plays a gently 'shushing' noise, called 'white noise', directly into the ear. This can help distract the brain from the sound of the tinnitus. A noise generator won't work for everyone, and some people find them annoying, so it is better to try one through your local tinnitus clinic, where you will get advice and support about using it.

Arnold

'I wear two hearing aids now; the one on my left ear helps my hearing, but the one on my right ear plays a sound called 'white noise' that

> masks my tinnitus. That helps a lot during the day. But at night, when I take my hearing aids out, the tinnitus seems louder than ever. If I wake up during the night I lie awake listening to it for hours – it's almost impossible to get back to sleep.'

It is best to get a noise generator through the NHS, as it can then be properly fitted. What is more important, it can be used with other techniques, for example as part of a Tinnitus Retraining Therapy (see below). But if this is not available in your area, it can be bought privately through a hearing aid dispenser, or even directly from a manufacturer, although this is not always satisfactory as there is less possibility of follow-up help.

Masking equipment to use at home

As well as devices that play sounds directly into the ear, it is possible to buy noise generators for use by the bedside or under the pillow to help someone sleep better. These are listed in a factsheet, *Sound and noise generators*, available from the RNID Tinnitus Helpline (address on page 142).

Cognitive therapy

This is a kind of psychological therapy in which the person learns to 'not hear' the sound of their tinnitus, by blocking the mental reactions which make the tinnitus intrusive or upsetting.

Their ear and brain are both involved in the process of hearing. Cognitive therapy teaches their brain to ignore the sounds coming from their ear.

Tinnitus Retraining Therapy

This is a therapy which combines a number of the techniques mentioned above. Gentle white noise is played over a period of time to make the person's brain less aware of tinnitus. Counselling and relaxation help them to be less bothered by their tinnitus, and to get less stressed by it. Finally, cognitive therapy helps the person to 'switch off' from the sound of their tinnitus.

We all know that some sounds are much more intrusive than others. To a parent, the sound of their baby crying seems like an alarm siren wailing in the ear, while someone else may hardly be aware of it at all. If we are in a situation we find frightening, we become acutely aware of sounds that might signal danger, which we simply don't hear most of the time. Tinnitus Retraining Therapy (TRT) uses this ability we have to 'switch off' sounds that are meaningless, so our brain is 're-trained' to ignore tinnitus.

Self-help

The best way to stop tinnitus becoming too bothersome is for the person you care for to keep busy, and keep their mind active. Exercise and relaxation can all help. People with tinnitus often find they get tremendous help and support from joining a self-help group. Apart from the relief of being with other people in the same situation, self-help groups are also a good source of information about what kinds of treatments are on offer in your area, and how effective they have been.

Many local groups are linked to the British Tinnitus Association. You can find out about groups in your area from the address on page 138, through the RNID Tinnitus Helpline (details on page 142) from your local library or audiology clinic.

How the carer can help

It can be hard for a carer to know whether it's best to offer support to someone by talking about their tinnitus, or whether it's better not to keep reminding them about it.

You should inform the person of the help that's available to them, but try not to badger them, even if you think they're being unreasonable or stubborn. This could simply make them feel more stressed – making their tinnitus even worse.

If someone is worried that tinnitus is a sign of something more serious, you can reassure them that this is not usually so. Tinnitus is annoying but harmless – it is very seldom a sign of anything more serious. Worrying about it does not help.

Be sensitive to the person's need for a certain amount of noise in their environment. Often people with tinnitus hate to be in a completely quiet room, as this makes their tinnitus seem much louder. A radio or some quiet music can make life tolerable for them. But of course if it's too loud, it could be intolerable to you!

For more *i*nformation

ⓘ The British Tinnitus Association (address on page 138) has a range of leaflets and information, including *Noises in the head or ears: all about tinnitus.*

ⓘ The British Tinnitus Association also produce a monthly magazine called *Quiet* for members (it costs £10 or less to join). They will also be able to put you in touch with the nearest local group.

ⓘ Contact the RNID Tinnitus Helpline (details on page 142) for advice, information, or just someone to talk to if things get desperate. The Helpline stocks more than 50 factsheets, books and relaxation tapes covering medical and complementary therapies.

ⓘ Other information available from RNID includes:
  - *A Layman's Guide to Tinnitus; Questions about Tinnitus* and the *Tinnitus Information Pack.*
  - *Online Tinnitus* is a newsletter for health professionals, local tinnitus groups and others concerned with tinnitus and hearing loss.
  - *One in Seven*, the RNID members' magazine, has a regular feature on tinnitus and a special tinnitus supplement.

Recruitment or loudness discomfort

People with a hearing loss sometimes suffer a condition called recruitment, also known as loudness discomfort, in which their ears seem to be unduly sensitive to loud sounds. It may seem to you that someone is just being awkward if one moment they say they can't hear you, and the next moment they say you are shouting too loud. But people with recruitment can only hear comfortably within quite a narrow range of sound volumes.

This may happen if the tiny hair cells in the inner ear are damaged and cannot pick up sounds easily. When the ear detects a sound it therefore very quickly calls on or 'recruits' all the remaining hair cells to help it listen. Thus any sound that is heard at all, is heard at once as being very loud or even painfully loud.

There is no cure for recruitment. Someone with recruitment also needs to have special care taken when a hearing aid is fitted, and to ask for an aid with automatic gain control (see page 47) so that the sound never gets uncomfortably loud. If the person you care for has an older model hearing aid, and complains of loudness discomfort, it may be time to take it back to the hearing aid clinic and ask for one with automatic gain control.

Chris

'I suffer severe recruitment, especially in noisy social situations. Then the noise and stress really set off my tinnitus. Family meals are difficult. In a big argument or discussion I just withdraw. It's easier to shut off. When they need me they shout, "MUM!" Parties are appalling. I have to put up with hours of tinnitus before I can even think of going to bed.'

For more *i*nformation

ℹ️ Hyperacusis, Recruitment and Loudness Discomfort by J W P Hazell. Available from the British Tinnitus Association or RNID (addresses on pages 138 and 142).

Dizziness

As well as hearing, our ears also govern our sense of balance. This is quite separate to the auditory system, and is controlled by fluid-filled organs in the inner ear called semicircular canals. People with damage to their inner ear may experience vertigo (dizziness) or balance problems. This can be associated with a hearing loss, but in many people with balance problems there is no hearing loss. Balance problems can be caused by a virus or poor blood supply, and these problems usually clear up of their own accord. However, dizziness caused by Menière's disease (see below) can recur over long periods of time.

For more *i*nformation

ⓘ The RNID Helpline (details on page 142) can provide further information about dizziness and balance problems, including the free leaflet, *Dizziness and balance problems.*

Menière's disease

Menière's disease is a rare disease of the inner ear that usually starts between the ages of 20 and 50, although it can occur at any age.

When pressure of fluids builds up in the inner ear, it causes an attack of vertigo, usually accompanied by sensorineural deafness and tinnitus. No one knows why this happens. In severe cases someone may have an attack once or twice a week, while other people may go for a year or more between attacks. It may mean that people cannot drive.

Flickering lights, strobe lighting, stripy or 'psychedelic' patterns, even light slanting through Venetian blinds, can all bring on an attack. Stress, too much salt, caffeine and alcohol have also been blamed.

Typically, an attack will include severe tinnitus and sickening vertigo lasting from a few minutes to a few hours. As the disease progresses, people may become imbalanced between attacks, which may spread out and become less frequent.

Many treatments have been tried, but no individual treatment has become established. If the person you care for has Menière's disease, it would be a good idea to discuss it with their GP as there might be a treatment that turns out to be suitable for them.

Judith

'It's a most distressing condition. Apart from the hearing loss you feel dreadful nausea, rather like you do with a migraine. Sometimes you can fall over with the vertigo, and instead of being sympathetic, people think you're drunk. Eventually it burns itself out, but sometimes the hearing loss is permanent.'

If you or the person you care for have been diagnosed with Menière's disease, you will find it helpful to join the Menière's Society, who can put you in touch with other people with the same condition and keep you up to date about research and treatments.

For more *i*nformation

i Contact the Menière's Society at the address on page 141.

i RNID Helpline (address on page 142) has a free factsheet about Menière's disease.

Deafblindness

Deafblindness is a very distressing condition, and one that many people imagine to be extremely rare. Unfortunately this is not so.

Although deafblindness among babies, children and young adults is now very unusual, it is increasing in the older population as people live longer. Both deafness and sight loss are a very common part of the ageing process. Almost all of us will experience a gradual deterioration of our sight and hearing as we get older. Thus it happens that someone with a hearing loss will gradually lose their eyesight as they get older, and someone who is blind or nearly blind will suffer the same gradual loss of hearing with age as the rest of us.

If the person you care for already has one sensory loss, and is now starting to lose another, they will need all the help and support you can give them. Firstly, they are quite likely to feel extremely depressed as their contact with the world seems to ebb away. Secondly, aids and assistance are available, but it may take energy and persistence to find out about what there is out there. They may feel too demoralised to make the effort.

Judith

'My Mum was deaf, then went blind in later life. She became very isolated. She wouldn't go out, because she couldn't see where she was going, and her sense of balance also went. They tried an operation, but it didn't work. It was quite traumatic for her. She was like that for five or six years before she died.'

People with hearing loss depend on many visual clues to help them to communicate. They may use sign language, or they may lipread, or they may carry a notebook and pencil around with them. Someone with both hearing and sight loss may find Braille helpful, but it takes some time to learn. The deafblind manual alphabet is a system of making letter shapes on the hand. This is the main way that hearing people communicate with deafblind people, and it is not difficult to learn.

Isolation is the main threat for deafblind people and you should do all you can to help the person you care for to feel less isolated.

113

Stuart

'It can be terrible for an elderly person living on their own. My mother is deafblind. She can't read a book; she can't watch television; she can speak, but communication takes time. My sister takes her out when she can. But even just sitting with her, holding her hand, makes her feel less alone.'

If the person you care for is becoming deafblind, here are some ways you can help:

■ Start learning the deafblind manual alphabet as soon as possible.

■ Find out which is their better sense, and make best use of it – make sure they have the best hearing aid and the best glasses possible. Audiology departments and hearing aid clinics are normally very sympathetic in this situation, and someone who is becoming deafblind should go straight to the top of the list, rather than having to wait several months.

■ Ask for an assessment by social services of their other needs, and discuss what aids may be available, for example a vibrating pager or a telephone with extra large keys and a volume amplifier (see Chapter 5, 'Managing at home', and Chapter 6, 'Using the telephone').

■ Ask the social services department about guide help schemes – people experienced in working with people with dual sensory loss who can assist the deafblind person on trips, such as visits to the shops or doctor.

■ Find out whether there are any deafblind groups in your area that the person you care for could join.

■ Try to spend some time with the deafblind person as often as you can and make an effort to communicate about things that are going on, in your family, in the neighbourhood, in the world, to break down that feeling of isolation.

■ Try to build a support network of family, friends and neighbours who will pop in and spend some time with the person you care for. Try to arrange an informal 'rota' so that there is someone to call round every day. Local churches, community groups, schools, often have 'befriending' schemes, where volunteers befriend lonely and isolated people. To find out about such schemes in your area, contact the local authority's social services department, or the local Council for Voluntary Service.

■ The local library will provide books with very large print and taped books.

For more *i*nformation

i Your local social services department will have a disability team or a sensory impairment team, who will be able to put you in touch with sources of help in your area.

i Your GP is the gateway to hospital services – make sure the special needs of the person you care for are noted, and that he or she goes to the top of the list.

i SENSE (National Deafblind and Rubella Organisation – address on page 143) is a voluntary organisation offering information, support and advice for people with sensory loss and their families.

i RNIB (address on page 141) can provide information and special services for deafblind people.

Alzheimer's disease and dementia

We all get forgetful as we get older, but some people suffer severe memory loss which affects their personality and their ability to live independently. This is sometimes called dementia. Alzheimer's disease is a condition in which some areas in the brain develop 'plaques', leading to memory loss. Another type of dementia affecting older people is called multi-infarct dementia, which is caused when tiny blood vessels in the brain burst.

People with a hearing loss are no more likely than anyone else in the population to suffer dementia. However, symptoms of hearing loss are often confused with symptoms of dementia, and that is why it is included in this chapter.

Someone with a hearing loss may find it difficult to follow a conversation. They may make answers which seem inappropriate, or they may ask about something which has just been said, because they didn't hear it properly the first time. However, this can give the impression that they have already forgotten what you were talking about only a few minutes ago, so you may think that they are losing their memory. It happens that people are wrongly diagnosed with Alzheimer's disease or dementia when in fact all they need is a good hearing aid.

On the other hand, someone with Alzheimer's disease or another kind of dementia may find it difficult to follow a conversation, because they keep on losing the thread of what has been said, but the carer may think that they simply cannot hear properly.

Julia

'My mother-in-law had Alzheimer's disease, but she was also going deaf. It was hard for us to work out whether her problems communicating were because she hadn't heard what was said, or because she kept forgetting. Then she went into a residential home, and they took away her glasses because they said she could hurt herself if she fell, and they took away her hearing aid because she didn't know how to use it. But for her it was terrible. It meant she was completely cut off, living in a world of her own.'

It's important that you and the doctor take the trouble to make sure the condition of the person you care for is properly diagnosed, and they are getting the most appropriate treatment.

For more *i*nformation

ℹ Contact the Alzheimer's Society at the address on page 137.

Depression

Pauline

'After Mum went completely deaf, she got really bad depression for a year or more. She just couldn't accept it. She kept asking, "Why me?" She would get angry and upset that she would never hear her grand-children's voices. There came a point when she said to herself, there's just no way I can carry on like this. Then she started to go to the deaf club. She met a little girl called Emily, who had hearing, but used sign language to communicate with her parents who were both deaf. Mum asked her how she had learnt sign language, and when she realised there were no books or anything to help her, Mum set about writing one. She and my sister wrote a children's 'ABC' guide to sign language. Well, that stirred up a lot of interest. It got into the book-shops, and into the newspapers, and before she knew it, a whole new world opened up for her.

'Now she's on the Community Health Council, and she's starting up a sign-language interpreters service, and she goes out to speak to schools and clubs. Nowadays you have to make an appointment to see her!'

It is not unusual for someone with hearing loss to become depressed. Someone who loses their hearing quite suddenly, like Pauline's mother, is likely to go through a period of 'mourning', rather like a bereavement, as they struggle to come to terms with their disability and to build a new life. They will have to learn to manage in a new and complex situation at a time when their morale and self-esteem are very low.

On the other hand, someone who loses their hearing gradually over a period of time may slip into depression as they gradually get cut off from social contact, and the long-term psychological consequences of hearing loss take their toll.

117

Albert

'I'm a pretty normal person, but I only communicate as far as I have to. When you can't hear, people treat you as if you're a bit stupid. Gradually, I found I was isolating myself from other people. I took up art – it was something I could do by myself. I didn't do it consciously, I just found myself becoming a loner.'

As a carer, you can help by reassuring the person you care for that their feelings are normal, and they will pass. It's sometimes hard not to get irritated or impatient with the person you care for if they don't follow your advice, or seem to you to be reacting disproportionately. That's a normal reaction – after all, carers are only human too! Understanding the feelings of the person you care for, and understanding your own reactions, can help you take a more philosophical view of what can be a very stressful situation.

If, like Albert, the person you care for is becoming isolated and lonely, then help them to build a new social world, perhaps through joining lipreading classes, or a Hard of Hearing Club. But remember, someone who is already lacking confidence will shrink at the thought of plunging into a completely new social situation. It is not enough to just give them information about groups and classes. You may need to go along with them a few times until they build up their confidence enough to go on their own, or at least make contact with someone already in the group or class who will take them under their wing.

Hearing Concern has a network of trained volunteer advisers who will visit someone at home, and provide sympathetic personal support to help someone come to terms with their hearing loss. The advisers are people who have a hearing loss themselves, who want to help others to cope with their loss. The service is free and completely confidential.

If the depression persists, and reassurance is not enough, then it is worth speaking to the person's GP about possible treatment for depression. Counselling and psychotherapy can help someone to come to terms with their loss, or the GP may offer anti-depressant medication.

For more *i*nformation

i Contact Hearing Concern address on page 140.

i Depression Alliance (address on page 139) can provide advice and information about depression and its treatment.

i The RNID Helpline (see page 142) is a good source of information for helping people coming to terms with their hearing loss.

9 Who can help?

There is a range of help available for people with hearing loss, but knowing where to find it can sometimes be a problem. Someone who has lost their confidence along with their hearing may not feel ready to go out and seek the support they are entitled to. The National Health Service, local authority social services and education departments, and the voluntary sector can all help in different ways. Unfortunately not all the services work together, so finding your way through the maze can be very confusing.

This chapter draws together an outline of the kinds of services that are provided for people with a hearing loss. But every local authority and every health trust has its own way of providing services, so the key to getting the best support for the person you care for is to find out who provides what in your area. To do this, you need to go through the 'gatekeeper' services. The family doctor is the 'gatekeeper' to access National Health Service provision, and the social services department is the 'gatekeeper' to access most other services. RNID and other voluntary organisations can give advice, information, and promote self help.

> ## Joan
>
> 'When Harry and I first got together, we were determined we wouldn't let his hearing loss get in the way, and we set out to find all the help there was. There is plenty of help if you look for it, but it's hard for someone who is deaf – they've got to be brave enough to go along, and they tend to hold back a bit. You have to feel your way when you talk to people – you don't know who can lipread, who can sign, who can fingerspell. But once you start getting involved, new doors open up for you.'

Help from the National Health Service

The National Health Service (NHS) provides treatment for the medical aspects of hearing loss. The 'gatekeeper' to NHS provision is the family doctor (GP). That means someone first has to go to the GP for 'primary care', and then if the GP thinks they need more help they will be referred for 'secondary care' to the local hospital. In some rare cases, for example when someone needs a highly specialised operation, they might be referred for 'tertiary care' to a regional or national centre that specialises in that particular treatment.

Although the NHS is mainly concerned with the medical aspects of hearing loss, there is an increasing understanding of the links between the body and the mind, and how hearing loss can have an impact on many other aspects of people's lives. Help with the psychological, emotional and social aspects of hearing loss is now often available through the NHS.

The GP's surgery or clinic (primary care)

Treatment offered by the GP or in a local clinic could include:

- diagnosing what's wrong with the ear(s);
- removing ear wax by syringing or by other means;

121

- antibiotics if an infection is suspected;
- treatment for depression or sleeping problems associated with hearing loss;
- referral to counselling or psychotherapy on the NHS;
- referral to ENT or audiology clinic for further hearing tests, treatment and hearing aids.

The hospital ENT department

Different hospitals are organised in different ways, but most people with a hearing problem will be referred either to an ENT (ear, nose and throat) clinic, or an audiology clinic. Hospital treatment could include:

- medication;
- surgery if this is recommended by the consultant;
- audiogram test to find out the degree and type of hearing loss;
- fitting a hearing aid;
- maintenance and repair of hearing aid;
- treatment for tinnitus;
- counselling or referral to psychological services;
- referral to another hospital or centre for specialised surgery.

Who's who at the audiology department

Ear, nose and throat consultant	Examines the ears and decides what treatment is necessary.
Audiometrist or audiologist	Tests hearing.
Audiologist or audiology technician	Fits the hearing aid; advises about use and maintenance.
Hearing therapist or audiology technician	Gives support and advice about coping with hearing loss.

There is more about getting help through the NHS in Chapter 4, 'Making the most of hearing aids'.

Help from social services

Social services provide support and practical help to people in the community to enable them to carry on living independently in their own homes.

Social services departments are organised in different ways throughout the country. They are usually divided into services for adults and services for children, with different teams of social workers responsible for each. There is often a specialist team of social workers to look after the needs of people with disabilities, and within this, there may be a social worker or a team of social workers dealing specifically with the needs of people with a hearing loss.

Although this organisation sounds quite complicated, getting through to the right person is usually easy. There will be a main switchboard number for the local authority social services department in the local telephone directory, and if you explain that you want advice about hearing loss, you will be put through to the right person.

Some people don't like the idea of contacting social services, because they think it is just for 'problem families' and they think they can manage within the family without 'running to others for help'. But this is a real pity. Social workers who specialise in hearing loss have a great interest and expertise in their subject, and can give you advice about all the practical aspects of caring for someone with hearing loss. They also know what is available locally, and can put you in touch with groups and organisations in your area. People who become social workers specialising in deafness and hearing loss often do so because of some personal or family experience, so their advice may be based on first-hand knowledge of the problems someone with hearing loss may face.

Merryl

'I grew up as a hearing child with parents who were both deaf. My first language was sign language. It was like growing up being bilingual. If anyone came to the door, I was the one who had to deal with them, even from a very early age. When one of my parents went to the doctor I would interpret for them – sometimes that was very stressful, if it was a delicate situation. When I grew up I knew I wanted to use my special insight and knowledge to help others in the same position. I worked as a sign language interpreter for a number of years, and then I trained as a social worker.'

If you contact social services on behalf of the person you care for, the first thing they will do is to carry out an assessment of the person's needs. The assessment looks at their degree of hearing loss and also their social situation – where they live, who is available to look after them, and any other health or mobility problems they have. If someone may be entitled to free equipment or services such as home care, then there may also be some questions about finances.

Moira

'"Assessment" is a very intimidating sort of word. I usually try to avoid it. When I contact someone, I never say I'm doing an assessment. I say "I'd just like to discuss your request …" or "I understand you're having difficulty with …" It's all very informal, and people often don't realise that's all an assessment is.'

When the social worker visits someone at home, he or she will not only assess the person's needs in relation to their hearing loss, but will also check whether they are eligible for home care, meals on wheels, personal care, any benefits they may not be claiming. The social worker also looks at the home – whether the toilet and washing facilities are suitable, whether the home is safe, whether there are urgent repairs that need to be done.

Moira

'People ring up and say, "All I want is a flashing doorbell", or something like that. But then when you meet them and explain all the other help they could be entitled to, they say, "Oh, I didn't think of that."'

Social services may be able to help with:

- an assessment of someone's needs;
- equipment to make living at home easier and safer (see Chapter 5, 'Managing at home'). This may be free or there may be a charge for it;
- advice about using a textphone – some local authorities provide a free textphone, usually for people with severe or profound hearing loss;
- other services such as meals on wheels, home help, personal care;
- information about grants to repair or insulate the home for people on a low income;
- information about social security benefits;
- contact with local groups and clubs for deaf or hard of hearing people;
- information about lipreading and sign language classes in your area;
- last but not least, help and support for carers (see below).

Help for carers

Looking after someone is a difficult and demanding job. Some carers, especially if they live with the person they care for, may find caring so stressful that they become ill themselves. If you are caring for someone who does not live with you, you have the constant worry whether they are all right. If they have hearing loss, even picking up the phone to give them a ring may not be easy.

Under the Carers and Disabled Children Act (2000) you are entitled to an assessment of your own needs as a carer. If you find caring is getting you down, contact your local social services department and ask for help – you are entitled to it by right.

If you are living with the person you care for, you should be able to get a break from caring from time to time. You may be able to get someone to sit in with the person you care for while you go out for a while during the day. Or you may be able to arrange for them to have a short stay in a residential or nursing home, so that you can have a break yourself, and maybe even go off on holiday. This kind of care is called respite care, and is available through your local authority social services department.

Getting help with caring isn't being selfish, it's being sensible. It means you can carry on caring for longer, and provide a better quality of care, because you are refreshed and relaxed.

Things you can do to make caring easier:

- Find out about respite care from the local authority.
- Join a carers' group or drop in at the carers' centre if there is one in your area. A burden shared is a burden halved.
- If you feel stress is affecting your health, talk to your GP. Going to see the doctor doesn't automatically mean 'being put on tranquillisers'. You may be able to see a counsellor or attend relaxation classes.
- Find out from the GP whether the person you care for is eligible for Attendance Allowance. If they are, you could be entitled to Invalid Care Allowance.
- Make time for yourself. Keep up with your own friends and interests.
- Look after your own health. Eat well, and take enough exercise.

Education and hearing loss

People who lose their hearing while they are still of school age will find that there is a great deal of support in the education system, either in special schools, or from special staff in mainstream schools. For people who lose their hearing when they are older, lipreading and sign language classes can be the gateways to a new world of communication. Some centres also run deaf awareness courses, or courses on understanding deafness. These classes are usually run by the education department of the local authority. Sometimes, however, they are run by individual colleges, education centres, community centres or audiology departments.

Different local authorities vary greatly in what they provide. To find out what is on offer in your area, try contacting:

- the main switchboard for the education department;
- individual colleges in your area;
- local community centres;
- the social services department (even if they don't provide any classes, they will know what's available);
- a local deaf association or hard of hearing club;
- Hearing Concern (see page 140 for contact details).

If you have no success, contact the Association of Teachers of Lipreading to Adults at the address on page 137.

Remember that joining a new class can be a very intimidating experience, especially for someone who has lost their confidence along with their deafness, so you may need to go along with them the first few times.

Help from the voluntary sector

The 'voluntary sector' is the name given to the huge range of charities, self-help organisations, special interest groups, drop-in centres and advice lines that are run neither by the Government nor by local authorities, but by independent groups of people with a special interest in a particular issue. Of course not everyone who works for these organisations is a volunteer, and most of them do get financial help from the Government or local authority, as well as through their own fundraising. They are independently managed, often by people with specialist knowledge, and they fill in the gaps left by the Government and local authorities (sometimes called the 'statutory sector').

For people with hearing loss, voluntary sector groups provide information, advice, helplines, home visits, social clubs and other activities. They also play an important role in campaigning for deaf and hard of hearing people, raising public awareness, and making sure that politicians take account of their needs.

The Royal National Institute for Deaf People

The Royal National Institute for Deaf People (RNID) is the largest organisation in the UK promoting the interests of deaf and hard of hearing people. It also has a campaigning role, working to raise awareness and change attitudes among the health service, politicians and the general public.

It publishes a range of helpful leaflets and factsheets and RNID Sound Advantage sells tried and tested equipment for deaf people at a reasonable price.

You or the person you care for can join RNID, and receive the bimonthly magazine *One in Seven*, which has articles, interviews, advice and information about the latest research, services, legislation, benefits, equipment and events. But even if you are not a member, you can still phone for information about:

- Equipment – everything from doorbells to induction loops.
- Communicating by telephone, textphone and Typetalk.
- Hearing aids – getting one from the NHS or buying one.
- Sign language – everything from learning sign language to finding an interpreter.
- Lipreading – classes or books to help you learn at home.
- Medical conditions and treatments – getting behind the medical jargon.
- Tinnitus – how to manage it.
- Self-help groups and social clubs.

You can contact RNID at the address on page 142. It has regional branches in Bristol, Belfast, Birmingham, Cardiff, Glasgow, London and Manchester.

Hearing Concern

Hearing Concern is a self-help charity whose members are mostly people with acquired hearing loss, who communicate through the spoken word, rather than through sign language. It tries to foster better communication between people who are hard of hearing and the hearing world, and it does this in two ways. First, it helps and advises hard of hearing people; second, it educates the hearing world about how to communicate with hard of hearing people.

Hearing Concern is particularly known for its network of Hard of Hearing Clubs, and trained volunteer advisers. These are usually hard of hearing people themselves, who have learned how to manage their hearing loss, and who visit hard of hearing people at home to give friendly, personal and confidential advice about any aspect of hearing loss and communication. They also run the Sympathetic Hearing Scheme, which encourages businesses and service providers to take into account the needs of customers and clients who have a hearing loss.

Help for hard of hearing people:

- telephone helpline (see page 140);
- social clubs and groups all over the country;
- quarterly *Hearing Concern* magazine;
- trained volunteer advisers, who will visit someone at home and can give support to first-time hearing aid users;
- promotes lipreading classes.

Educating the public:

- Sympathetic Hearing Scheme (see pages 80–81);
- training for volunteers, professionals and organisations;
- training for lipreading teachers.

You can contact Hearing Concern at the address on page 140.

Local groups and clubs

Joining a deaf club or a hard of hearing association can open up a whole new world of social contacts and activities for someone who has a hearing loss. They will find people to talk with, go out with, go on holiday with, and they will find support and friendship from others who are in the same situation. It is important for the person you care for to find a place where they can feel comfortable and included in the social scene.

Deaf clubs tend to be more popular with people who have grown up in the Deaf Community, and who communicate through sign language, though people who use a hearing aid or communicate through lipreading are welcome too.

Hard of hearing associations tend to serve those who grew up in the hearing community and lost their hearing later in life, and who communicate through speech and lipreading. Most older people fall into this group.

You can find out about local groups and clubs in your area from the social services department, the public library, or the hearing aid clinic. The person you care for may be more willing to go along if you accompany them the first few times.

Benefits for people with a hearing loss

Social security benefits are the way we as a society provide for ourselves in times of need. There is nothing to be ashamed of in claiming a benefit, any more than there would be in drawing a pension. If you think the person you care for could qualify for one of the benefits listed below, there is nothing to be lost and much to be gained in applying.

Claims for benefits are dealt with by the Benefits Agency. You can get the address for your local Benefits Agency office by asking at a local library or post office, or you can look in the telephone directory where it will be listed under 'Benefits Agency' or 'social security'. You can contact your local office by telephone, by letter or by going in person. If the person you care for has difficulties getting out, they can ask for a visiting officer to come to their home.

For advice and information about disability benefits, you can telephone the National Benefit Enquiry Line on 0800 88 22 00; textphone 0800 24 33 55. Enquiry Line staff can also complete forms for you over the phone for benefits such as Attendance Allowance and Disability Living Allowance (see below).

Disability Living Allowance

Someone who is below the age of 65 may be able to claim Disability Living Allowance. This is a social security benefit to help with the extra costs of disability. It is not dependent on the person's income or savings and will not normally affect any other benefits or pensions they are receiving.

To claim, obtain a special claim pack from your local Benefits Agency office.

Incapacity Benefit

This is a benefit for people below pension age who cannot work as a result of illness or disability. To qualify for this benefit, someone's incapacity for work has to be assessed, and they have to have paid National Insurance contributions.

To claim, obtain a special claim pack from your local Benefits Agency office.

Attendance Allowance

This allowance is for people aged 65 or over who need to be looked after in some way, for example helped with washing, getting dressed, eating, using the toilet, or having someone to watch over them in case they hurt themselves. Someone who has a hearing loss will not normally qualify for Attendance Allowance unless they have some other illness or disability as well. However, if the person you care for has some other condition as well as hearing loss, then they should ask at the local Benefits Agency office whether they would be eligible for Attendance Allowance. It does not depend on the person's income or savings and is not taxable.

To claim, obtain a special claim pack from your local Benefits Agency office.

Invalid Care Allowance

This is a benefit for carers who spend 35 hours a week or more looking after someone. The person they look after has to be claiming the care component of Disability Living Allowance at the middle or higher rates or Attendance Allowance.

To claim, obtain a special claim pack from your local Benefits Agency office.

Industrial Injuries Disablement Benefit

Someone who lost their hearing through working in a noisy occupation or through an accident at work may be able to claim this benefit. It is not dependent on income or savings and the person you care for may be able to claim even if they are still working.

To find out more about this benefit, contact your local Benefits Agency office and ask for leaflet NI207.

Compensation for industrial deafness

If you think the person you care for may have lost their hearing as a result of their job, they may be entitled to compensation.

Contact their trade union or a solicitor who specialises in industrial injuries to find out how to claim.

War pension

Someone who lost their hearing as a result of service during the war may be able to apply for a special war pension. They will have to have a hearing test and answer questions about how and when the hearing loss occurred. The pension is tax free, and is not means tested.

People may qualify if they lost their hearing as a result of service:

- in HM armed forces;
- in Polish Forces under British Command or Polish Resettlement Forces in the 1939–45 war;
- the Civil Defence Volunteer corps in the 1939–45 war;
- the merchant navy or coastguard service or auxiliary services.

OR if they lost their hearing:

- as a result of enemy action;
- as a result of detention by the enemy.

To find out more, and to make a claim, telephone the War Pensions Helpline: 01253 858 858.

For more *information*

ⓘ Contact RNID (address on page 142) or Hearing Concern (address on page 140).

ⓘ For information about most social security benefits, contact your local Benefits Agency office (the number is in your local telephone directory).

ⓘ War Pensions Helpline: 01253 858 858.

ⓘ For advice and information about disability benefits, telephone the Department of Social Security National Benefit Enquiry Line for disabled people: 0800 88 22 00; textphone 0800 24 33 55 (8.30am to 6.30pm weekdays; 9am to 1pm Saturdays). Staff can also complete forms over the phone for benefits such as Attendance Allowance and Disability Living Allowance. Calls are free.

i *Finding and paying for residential and nursing home care* and *Choices for the carer of an elderly relative*, both written by Marina Lewycka and available from Age Concern (see page 147).

i Age Concern Factsheet 18 *A brief guide to money benefits* and Factsheet 34 *Attendance Allowance and Disability Living Allowance* (see page 150).

i *Your Rights: A guide to money benefits for older people* is an annual guide to the State benefits available to older people, published by Age Concern (see page 148).

Glossary

Audiogram Graph showing measurement of hearing levels.

BAHA Bone-anchored hearing aid.

BiCROS Bicontralateral Routing of Signals (see page 46).

BTE Behind-the-ear hearing aid.

BW Body-worn hearing aid.

Conductive deafness Deafness caused by sound waves being unable to pass through the outer or middle ear, possibly due to blockage or infection.

CROS Contralateral Routing of Signals (see page 46).

dBHL Decibel Hearing Level – used to measure sound.

Deaf Usually means someone is profoundly or severely deaf.

Hard of hearing Describes someone who can understand so long as the speaker speaks clearly.

Hearing impaired A broad term which can cover the whole range of hearing disabilities; usually used in medical or educational settings.

Hearing loss A broad term covering the whole range of hearing disabilities.

Hertz A measure of frequency.

Induction loop Magnetic loop that transmits sounds within its scope to hearing aid or listening device.

Infrared system Sound transmitter that works by infrared light.

ITC In-the-canal hearing aid.

ITE In-the-ear hearing aid.

Listening device Amplification system linking TV or radio to headphones.

Menière's disease A rare disease of the inner ear that damages both the hearing and balance parts of the ear.

Minicom Brand name of textphone (see below).

Post-lingual deafness When someone has lost their hearing after learning speech.

Pre-lingual deafness When someone is born deaf or becomes deaf before learning to talk.

Profoundly deaf A person who is profoundly deaf has little or no hearing at all.

Sensorineural deafness Deafness caused by damage to the cochlea or the auditory nerve.

Stetoclip Small headphones like those of a stethoscope.

Textphone Equipment that enables deaf people to type conversations down a telephone line.

Tinnitus Name given to sounds in a person's head which have no apparent source.

Typetalk Telephone relay service linking textphone users with people using ordinary voice phones.

Useful addresses

Alzheimer's Society
Gordon House
10 Greencoat Place
London SW1P 1PH
Tel: 020 7306 0606
Helpline: 0845 300 0336

Information, support and advice about caring for someone with Alzheimer's disease.

Association of Teachers of Lipreading to Adults (ATLA)
PO Box 506
Hanley
Stoke on Trent ST2 9RE
Tel: 01709 815516
Email: atla@lipreading.org.uk

To find out about lipreading classes in your area.

Benefit Enquiry Line and Form Completion
Tel: 0800 88 22 00 (a free call) 8.30am–6.30pm weekdays, 9am–1pm Saturdays.
Textphone: 0800 24 33 55

For advice and information about disability benefits. Staff can also complete forms over the phone for benefits such as Attendance Allowance and Disability Living Allowance.

British Deaf Association
1–3 Worship Street
London EC2A 2AB
Tel: 020 7588 3520

Information and social support for deaf people.

British Red Cross
9 Grosvenor Crescent
London SW1X 7EJ
Tel: 020 7235 5454

Can loan home aids for disabled people. Local branches.

British Tinnitus Association
4th Floor, White Building
Fitzalan Square
Sheffield S1 2AZ
Tel: 0114 279 6600
Fax: 0114 279 6222
Freephone enquiry line: 0800 018 0527

Advice and support for people with tinnitus. Contact details for local support groups.

Carers National Association
20–25 Glasshouse Yard
London EC1A 4JT
Tel: 020 7490 8818 (1–4pm weekdays)

Information and advice if you are caring for someone. Can put you in touch with other carers and carers' groups in your area.

Citizens Advice Bureau
Listed in local telephone directories, or in the *Yellow Pages* under 'Counselling and advice'. Other local advice centres may also be listed.

For advice on legal, financial and consumer matters. A good place to turn to if you don't know where to go for help or advice on any subject.

Council for the Advancement of Communication with Deaf People (CACDP)
Durham University Science Park
Block 4
Stockton Road
Durham DH1 3UZ
Tel: 0191 383 1155

Fax: 0191 383 7914
Textphone: 0191 383 7915
E-mail: durham@cacdp.demon.co.uk

Research and projects that promote communication for deaf and hard-of-hearing people with the wider community.

Counsel and Care
Lower Ground Floor
Twyman House
16 Bonny Street
London NW1 9PG
Tel: 020 7485 1566 (10am–4pm)

Advice for older people and their families; can sometimes give grants to help people remain at home, or return to their home.

Crossroads Care
10 Regent Place
Rugby
Warwickshire CV21 2PN
Tel: 01788 573653

For a care attendant to come and look after your relative at home.

Department of Health
PO Box 410
Wetherby
LS23 7LN
Fax: 01937 845 381

For copies of the leaflet How to use your hearing aid.

Depression Alliance
35 Westminster Bridge Road
London SE1 7JB
Tel: 020 7633 0557

Support and information for people experiencing depression.

Disabled Living Foundation
380–384 Harrow Road
London W9 2HU
Tel: 020 7289 6111
Information about aids to help you cope with a disability.

The Forest Bookshop
Warehouse
8 Crucible Court
Coleford
Glos GL16 8RF
Tel: 01594 833858 (voice and textphone)
Fax: 01594 833446
E-mail: deafbooks@forestbooks.com
Website: www.ForestBooks.com

Specialise in books, videos and CD-ROMs about deafness and deaf issues. A mail order catalogue is available.

Hearing Aid Council
Witan Court
305 Upper Fourth Street
Central Milton Keynes MK9 1EH
Tel: 01908 235700
Information about all aspects of hearing aids.

Hearing Concern
7–11 Armstrong Road
London W3 7JL
Tel: 020 8743 1110 (admin)
Fax: 020 8742 9043
Textphone: 020 8742 9151
E-mail: hearingconcern@hearingconcern.com
Helpline: 0845 0744 600 (voice and textphone)
Website: www.hearingconcern.com

Advice about communication and support at home for those who have lost their hearing. Also promote the Sympathetic Hearing Scheme to encourage better understanding and communication within the wider community.

Hearing Dogs for Deaf People
The Training Centre
London Road
Lewknor
Oxon OX49 5RY
Tel: 01844 353898 (voice and textphone)

To find out more about how hearing dogs can help those with hearing loss.

Lipservice
Milton House
Stratfield Saye
Reading RG7 2BT

Information and videos about communication and lipreading.

Menière's Society
98 Maybury Road
Woking
Surrey GU21 5HX
Tel: 01483 740597

A support group for people with Menière's disease and their families.

Relatives and Residents Association
5 Tavistock Place
London WC1H 9SN
Helpline: 020 7916 6055 (10am–4.30pm weekdays)

Advice for relatives and friends of people in care homes; work to improve the quality of care in care homes.

Royal National Institute for the Blind (RNIB)
224 Great Portland Street
London W1W 5AA
Tel: 020 7388 1266
Helpline: 0345 669 999 (9am–5pm weekdays)

Advice, information and support for all aspects of sight loss.

The Royal National Institute for Deaf People (RNID)
19–23 Featherstone Street
London EC1Y 8SL
Tel: 020 7296 8000
Textphone: 020 7296 8001
Website: www.rnid.org.uk

Advice, information, social support, and an extensive list of publications, covering all aspects of hearing loss. See page 144 for more about RNID.

RNID Helpline
PO Box 16464
London EC1Y 8TT
Helpline: 0808 808 0123
Helpline textphone: 0808 808 9000
E-mail: helpline@rnid.org.uk

RNID Sound Advantage
1 Metro Centre
Welbeck Way
Peterborough PE2 7UH
Tel: 01733 361199
Fax: 01733 361161
Textphone: 01733 238020
E-mail: solutions@rnid.org.uk
Website: www.rnid.org.uk

Information about products specially designed to help people with hearing loss.

RNID Tinnitus Helpline
Tel: 0808 808 6666 (10am–3pm weekdays)
Textphone: 0808 808 0007
Fax: 0115 978 5012
Website: www.rnid.org.uk
E-mail: tinnitushelpline@rnid.org.uk

SENSE (National Deafblind and Rubella Organisation)
11–13 Clifton Terrace
London N4 3SR
Tel: 020 7272 7774

Support and advice for people who have dual sensory loss.

Social Security
For information about most social security benefits, contact your local Benefits Agency office (the number is in your local telephone directory).

Sympathetic Hearing Scheme
See *Hearing Concern*

Typetalk
PO Box 284
Liverpool L69 3UZ
Tel: 0800 7311 888
Textphone: 0800 500 888
Fax: 0151 709 8119

A telephone service for people with hearing loss who have a textphone, which enables them to communicate with hearing people through a Typetalk operator.

War Pensions Helpline
War Pensions Agency
Norcross
Blackpool FY5 3WP
Tel: 0800 169 2277 (Monday–Thursday 8.15am–5.15pm, Friday 8.15am–4.30pm).

For general advice on war pensions.

About The Royal National Institute for Deaf People (RNID)

The Royal National Institute for Deaf People (RNID) is the largest charity representing the 8.7 million deaf and hard of hearing people in the UK. As a membership charity, it aims to achieve a radically better quality of life for deaf and hard of hearing people. It does this in the following ways:

- Campaigning and lobbying to change laws and government policies.
- Providing information and raising awareness of deafness, hearing loss and tinnitus.
- Training courses and consultancy on deafness and disability.
- Communication services including sign language interpreters.
- Training of interpreters, lipspeakers and speech-to-text operators.
- Seeking lasting change in education for deaf children and young people.
- Employment programmes to help deaf people into work.
- Residential and community services for deaf people with special needs.
- Typetalk, the national telephone relay service for deaf and hard of hearing people.
- Equipment and products for deaf and hard of hearing people.
- Social, medical and technical research.

See page 142 for RNID contact details.

About Age Concern

Caring for someone with a hearing loss is one of a wide range of publications produced by Age Concern England, the National Council on Ageing. Age Concern cares about all older people and believes later life should be fulfilling and enjoyable. For too many this is impossible. As the leading charitable movement in the UK concerned with ageing and older people, Age Concern finds effective ways to change that situation.

Where possible, we enable older people to solve problems themselves, providing as much or as little support as they need. Our network of 1,400 local groups and organisations, supported by 250,000 volunteers, provides community-based services such as lunch clubs, day centres and home visiting.

Nationally, we take a lead role in campaigning, parliamentary work, policy analysis, research, specialist information and advice provision, and publishing. Innovative programmes promote healthier lifestyles and provide older people with opportunities to give the experience of a lifetime back to their communities.

Age Concern is dependent on donations, covenants and legacies.

Age Concern England
1268 London Road
London SW16 4ER
Tel: 020 8765 7200
Fax: 020 8765 7211

Age Concern Scotland
113 Rose Street
Edinburgh EH2 3DT
Tel: 0131 220 3345
Fax: 0131 220 2779

Age Concern Cymru
4th Floor
1 Cathedral Road
Cardiff CF1 9SD
Tel: 029 2037 1566
Fax: 029 2039 9562

Age Concern Northern Ireland
3 Lower Crescent
Belfast BT7 1NR
Tel: 028 9032 5729
Fax: 028 9023 5497

Other books in this series

The Carers Handbook series has been written for the families and friends of older people. It guides readers through key care situations and aims to help readers make informed, practical decisions. All the books in the series:

- are packed full of detailed advice and information;
- offer step-by-step guidance on the decisions that need to be taken;
- examine all the options available;
- are full of practical checklists and case studies;
- point you towards specialist help;
- guide you through the social services maze;
- help you to draft a personal plan of action;
- are fully up to date with recent guidelines and issues;
- draw on Age Concern's wealth of experience.

Already published:

Caring for someone with arthritis
Jim Pollard
£6.99 0–86242–266–3

Caring for someone with diabetes
Marina Lewycka
£6.99 0–86242–282–5

Caring for someone with a heart problem
Toni Battison
£6.99 0–86242–252–3

Caring for someone with an alcohol problem
Mike Ward
£6.99 0–86242–227–2

Caring for someone who has had a stroke
Philip Coyne with Penny Mares
£6.99 0–86242–264–7

Caring for someone at a distance
Julie Spencer-Cingöz
£6.99 0–86242–228–0

Choices for the carer of an elderly relative
Marina Lewycka
£6.99 0–86242–263–9

Finding and paying for residential and nursing home care
Marina Lewycka
£6.99 0–86242–261–2

Caring for someone who has dementia
Jane Brotchie
£6.99 0–86242–259–0

Caring for someone who is dying
Penny Mares
£6.99 0–86242–260–4

The Carer's Handbook: What to do and who to turn to
Marina Lewycka
£6.99 0–86242–262–0

If you would like to order any of these titles, please write to the address below, enclosing a cheque or money order for the appropriate amount (plus £1.95 p&p) made payable to Age Concern England. Credit card orders may be made on 0870 44 22 044 (for individuals/members of the public); 0870 44 22 120 (AC federation/organisations and institutions); Fax: 01626 323318

Age Concern Books
PO Box 232
Newton Abbot
Devon TQ12 4XQ

Publications from Age Concern Books

Your Rights: A guide to money benefits for older people
Sally West

A highly acclaimed annual guide to the State benefits available to older people. It contains current information on Income Support, Housing Benefit and retirement pensions, among other matters, and provides advice on how to claim.

For more information, please telephone 0870 44 22 044

Better Health in Retirement
Dr Anne Roberts

A little attention to your body's changing needs and some knowledge of how to deal with common illnesses can lead to a long and healthy retirement. Written in non-medical language, this book gives practical, expert advice and information to help everyone keep as healthy as possible in later life. Topics include:

- common illnesses of later life
- using the health service
- complementary medicines
- help for older carers

This book also provides clear guidance on areas such as depression, sleeping well and relaxation techniques. Positive and upbeat, this book will equip readers with all of the information needed to take charge of their own health.

£6.99   0–86242–251–5

Age Concern Information Line

Age Concern produces over 40 comprehensive factsheets designed to answer many of the questions older people – or those advising them – may have, on topics such as:

- finding and paying for residential and nursing home care
- money benefits
- finding help at home
- legal affairs
- making a will
- help with heating
- raising income from your home
- transfer of assets

Age Concern offers a factsheet subscription service that presents all the factsheets in a folder, together with regular updates throughout the year. The first year's subscription currently costs £70. Single copies, up to a maximum of five, are available free on receipt of an sae.

To order your FREE factsheet list, phone 0800 00 99 66 (a free call) or write to:

Age Concern
FREEPOST (SWB 30375)
Ashburton
Devon TQ13 7ZZ

Index

alarms 60
  door 58, 59–60
  smoke 60–61
allowances *see* benefits
Alzheimer's disease 115–116
assessments, social security 124, 126
Attendance Allowance 131–132
audiograms 10, 11, 39

background noise, cutting down 24–25, 65
banks 79, 88–90
benefits, social security 130–134
blindness *see* deafblindness
building societies 79, 88–90
bus travel 96–97

carers 5, 39, 77, 84
  help for 125–126
churches 90–91
cinemas 77, 93–94
clubs, deaf 130
cochlea, the 17, 18, 19, 21
cochlear implants 46–47
communication 22–24, 81–82
  and background noise 24–25, 65
  by fingerspelling 32
  by lipreading 25–29, 32
  obstructions to 31
  and planning ahead 23, 78–79

by sign language 29–31, 32
by Sign Supported English 31
and Sympathetic Hearing Scheme 80–81
see also induction loops

dangers 99–100
deafblindness 112–115
deafness *see* hearing loss
decibels 10
dementia 115–116
depression 117–119
Disability Living Allowance 131
discrimination 100
diseases: and hearing loss 21
dizziness/vertigo 17, 102, 111
  see also Menière's disease
doctors *see* GPs
dogs, hearing 65–67
door alarms/bells 58, 59–60

ear, the 16, 17, 18
education: and hearing loss 126–127
ENT clinics 10, 38, 39–40, 122
eustachian tube, the 16, 17, 20

fingerspelling 32
furnishings 25, 58–59

'glue ear' 17, 20
GPs 9–10, 82–85